Women & Psychosis

Psychoanalytic Studies: Clinical, Social, and Cultural Contexts

Series Editor

Michael O'Loughlin, Adelphi University

Mission Statement

Psychoanalytic Studies seeks psychoanalytically informed works addressing the implications of the location of the individual in clinical, social, cultural, historical, and ideological contexts. Innovative theoretical and clinical works within psychoanalytic theory and in fields such as anthropology, education, and history are welcome. Projects addressing conflict, migrations, difference, ideology, subjectivity, memory, psychiatric suffering, physical and symbolic violence, power, and the future of psychoanalysis itself are welcome, as are works illustrating critical and activist applications of clinical work. See https://rowman.com/Action/SERIES/LEX/LEXPS for a list of advisory board members.

Titles in the Series

Women & Psychosis: Multidisciplinary Perspectives, edited by Marie Brown and Marilyn Charles

Psychoanalysis from the Indian Terroir: Emerging Themes in Culture, Family, and Childhood in India, edited by Manasi Kumar, Anup Dhar, and Anurag Mishra

A Three-Factor Model of Couples Psychotherapy: Projective Identification, Level of Couple Object Relations, And Omnipotent Control, by Robert Mendelsohn

Women & Psychosis

Multidisciplinary Perspectives

Edited by Marie Brown and Marilyn Charles

LEXINGTON BOOKS
Lanham • Boulder • New York • London

Published by Lexington Books
An imprint of The Rowman & Littlefield Publishing Group, Inc.
4501 Forbes Boulevard, Suite 200, Lanham, Maryland 20706
www.rowman.com

6 Tinworth Street, London SE11 5AL

British Library Cataloguing in Publication Information Available

Library of Congress Cataloging-in-Publication Data
Names: Brown, Marie, 1981- editor. | Charles, Marilyn, editor.
Title: Women & psychosis : multidisciplinary perspectives / edited by Marie Brown and Marilyn Charles.
Other titles: Women and psychosis
Description: Lanham, Md. : Lexington Books, [2019] | Series: Psychoanalytic studies: Clinical, social, and cultural contexts | Includes bibliographical references and index.
Identifiers: Identifiers: LCCN 2018059701 (print) | LCCN 2018061509 (ebook) | ISBN 9781498591928 (electronic) | ISBN 9781498591911 (cloth) ISBN 9781498591935 (pbk)
Subjects: LCSH: Women--Psychology. | Psychoses.
Classification: LCC HQ1206 (ebook) | LCC HQ1206 .W8676 2019 (print) | DDC 155.3/33--dc23
LC record available at https://lccn.loc.gov/2018059701

Contents

Preface   vii
Marie Brown

Introduction   1
Marie Brown and Marilyn Charles

I: WOMEN & PSYCHOSIS IN ARTS & CULTURE   **9**

1   Women and Madness in Context   11
Marilyn Charles

2   Explicate or Relate: Recognizing and Differentiating Literary
Madwomen   37
Helen DeVinney

3   Stories   59
Berta Britz

II: WOMEN, PSYCHOSIS & THE BODY   **79**

4   Snakes in the Crib: Psychosocial Factors in Postpartum Psychosis   81
Marie Brown

5   Disordered Eating and Distorted Thinking in Women: A
Continuum in Objectification in Anorexia and Psychosis   109
Jessica Arenella

III: WOMEN, PSYCHOSIS & SPIRITUALITY   **123**

6   Mystics, Witches, or Hysterics?: The Therapeutic Stakes When
Spirituality Becomes a Symptom   125
Liane F. Carlson

7   From Sick to Gifted: Discovering Shamanic Illness   149
    Gogo Ekhaya Esima

**IV: PSYCHIATRIC PERSPECTIVES ON WOMEN &
    PSYCHOSIS**   **159**

8   Psychosis in Women: A Perspective from Psychiatry   161
    Simone Ciufolini and Nicola Byrne

9   Schizophrenia in Women as Compared to Men: Theories to
    Help Explain the Difference   187
    Mary V. Seeman

Index   203

About the Editors and Contributors   211

Preface

Marie Brown

"What is the history of the idea to have this meeting?"

I grew up in a home marked by alcoholism, chaos, and domestic violence. I felt very alone in my suffering, my family members existing together but as isolated islands. I didn't have anyone I could talk to about what was going on. As a result, by the time I reached early adolescence, the world felt like a strange place. Periodically, I would be talking to someone or just sitting in class, and it was suddenly as if the lights were turned up really bright. I could see things in hyper-reality. It was as if—without warning—I had become aware of "The Truth of Things," viewing my surroundings with crystal clear vision. It caused me to feel alienated from other people and estranged from my environment. People's bodies looked fleshy and weird; they looked like apes that could talk, smile, and laugh. Everyone was moving together and playing along in a game that seemed absurd. Did they notice that I was somehow different? During these experiences, I would become filled with a sense of unnamable terror and a fear of mental (or even spiritual) fragmentation. I would look down at my hands and feel a disconnection from my body. My body seemed to operate on its own, a type of machine or automaton. I would move my hand and be terrified by the clarity with which I was experiencing it.

Alone in my bed at night, I would feel painful shocks of electricity shoot up from the sides of my neck into my head. The electricity was simultaneously a buzzing sound and a sensation—a horrible, searing sensation. I hypothesized that the shocks were coming from my parents—they had invented some type of machine to torture me at night by sending invisible rays into my head. I worried that the shocks were intended to warp my brain. I was scared that it would result in fundamental changes to my personality. I threw pillows over my head in an attempt to block the rays of the machine. In the morning, I would forget that it had ever happened.

I coped with my profound feelings of sadness, anxiety, and alienation by developing a rich fantasy world. I became closely connected to another girl named Sara. She played a leading role in my fantasy life. When we walked outside together, the backyard took on an otherworldly, mystical quality. It was like we were walking into another dimension. We had secret names in that other dimension and were considered to be profoundly special and magical beings there. I became heavily interested in the occult. I would go to the library and pour over books about the Salem witch trials, the *Malleus Malefi-carum*, and modern Wicca. I loved reading about witches and would imagine them naked, sneaking off into the woods at night, painting their bodies, and dancing wildly around raging bonfires. I felt like Sara and I were witches, keepers of supernatural abilities that other people could not understand. We would burn candles together and chant. I felt deeply powerful.

Once when I was at Sara's house I somehow ended up inside her shed alone. I don't remember how I got there, but I do remember that once inside I lost the ability to move my body. I had become trapped in a fetal position, hidden under a table. I had a hyper-awareness of my body being locked in place. The sensation was not entirely new to me. I had previously experienced moments where I lost the ability to move. If my parents were arguing, my body would sometimes take on a life of its own and stiffen up like a statue—even my eyes would become transfixed and immovable. Years later, I came across a quote by Wittgenstein and felt that it described me; he spoke about the remainder of pain, even after turning to stone.

I only have fragments of memories from that day in Sara's shed. I remember it being winter time, the ground covered in a light dusting of snow, but for some reason I wasn't wearing any shoes or jacket. I remember wearing a short, bright red cheongsam—a traditional Chinese dress—embroidered with golden dragons. I had some sort of outside awareness that people were searching for me. I could almost see the helicopters flying overhead, but I was still unable to move—my arms and legs stiffly bent in place. I don't know how long I was there, but at some point, a K-9 dog came and began sniffing at my neck. Shortly after, the police arrived. The shock of their flashlights and uniforms brought me back into my body and, although dazed, I was able to stand up and walk. I remember my mom helping me put my shoes and backpack on. It was heavy with textbooks. The next thing I remember after that was being brought to CPEP—the Comprehensive Psychiatric Emergency Program.

The CPEP was a bizarre experience. I remember pacing the waiting room in my short red cheongsam. An older man, another patient waiting to be seen, sneered at me "Why are you wearing that dress? Don't you know its winter?" I became profoundly aware of how short the dress was and how inappropriately sexual I must have looked to others. I yanked at the hem of my dress, trying to pull it down over my knees. "That's why you're in here—because of wearing dresses like that!" he shouted. I must have been about twelve or thirteen years old.[1]

I was brought to a back room filled with people. In my memory, they are all men wearing white lab coats. They shined a bright light in my face and I was placed under a gigantic magnifying glass. I realize now that must not have been literal, but it certainly appears that way in my mind, even today. I remember them firing questions at me, "What day of the week is it?" "Are you hearing voices?" "Who is the current president?" I can't remember what happened next, but after many hours, I was released. In the car home, my mom said to me that I didn't belong there. I didn't feel like I did either.

In Open Dialogue—a psychotherapeutic approach for helping people who are experiencing psychosis, their families, and social networks—all meetings start with the same question: "What is the history of the idea to have this meeting?" In the spirit of feminism, and the second-wave ethos of "the personal is the political," I decided to open *Women & Psychosis* with a fragment of my own experience. It would be disingenuous to say that I have ever experienced a "psychotic break." However, I do feel that my own atten-uated experiences have deeply informed the way that I currently understand what is commonly referred to as "psychosis." I do not believe that my experi-ences were the result of brain disease per se, but instead natural responses to what was going on around me—experiences with symbolic or metaphorical meanings that could not be expressed with words. No, my parents did not build a machine to shock my brain at night—but on another level, I *was* being "tortured" by their constant fighting and by my father's physical vio-lence. Perhaps an unconscious part of me worried about how it would affect me later in life—would it forever change me? Warp my personality? My body freezing in place could be understood as a physical manifestation of what I was unable to fully comprehend at the time—that I was stuck in my situation as it was, unable to find a way to move beyond it.

It is not surprising to me that my strange experiences with the world began in early adolescence—the point in time that one shifts from "being a girl" to "becoming a woman." In thinking about my situation through the lens of French psychoanalysts Davoine and Gaudillière (2004), I can recog-nize that overlaying the "little history" of my personal trauma growing up, was the "Big History" of becoming a woman in a culture that, at best, was ambivalent toward women. Looking back, perhaps it is not surprising that I turned to witches—their otherworldly and powerful femininity a stark contrast to the way that I experienced the real women around me. However, those witches paid deeply for their powers. In college, the witches were replaced by feminists—Sojourner Truth, Simone de Beauvoir, Audre Lorde, Luce Irigaray, Julia Kristeva, Virginia Woolf, Kathleen Hanna, bell hooks,

Patricia Hill Collins, Susan B. Anthony, Judith Butler, Inga Muscio, Mary Wollstonecraft. It is from this history that the idea for *Women & Psychosis* came about.

So why is it important to create a book about women and psychosis? From the ecstatic visions of medieval female mystics to Charlotte Perkins Gilman's yellow wallpaper, women have historically had an interesting relationship with psychosis. Located at a challenging sociopolitical intersection, women experiencing psychosis can be considered to bear the burden of two "discredited identities" (Goffman, 1963)—that of their gender and that of their psychiatric status. These two signifiers are often seen as interacting in complex ways. For example, feminist writer Phyllis Chesler (1972) discusses the fashion in which the diagnosis of "schizophrenia" has often served a punitive function for women experiencing "sex-role alienation" or "the inability to fully act out the conditioned female role" (p. 56). Similarly, Jane Ussher (1992) sees the "madness of women" not as biologically derived "mental illness" but as a sane response to an oppressive patriarchal world. Although important contributions in their own right, this kind of critical engagement has often failed to connect the everyday lived experience of women with psychosis and has perhaps failed to sufficiently acknowledge the fact of human suffering.

From the perspective of psychiatric research, women's experiences of psychosis have been found to be qualitatively different from those of their male counterparts (Seeman, 2012). "Auditory hallucinations" (or "hearing voices") are more common in women diagnosed with schizophrenia, than in men (Rector & Seeman, 1992). However, women diagnosed with schizophrenia are found to be less inclined toward social withdrawal (Morgan, Castle, & Jablensky, 2008), suggesting that they are more likely to maintain their social obligations as partners and mothers despite their psychotic symptoms. Women are also more likely to experience psychotic symptoms connected to shifts in their reproductive cycles, including phenomena such as menstrual and postpartum psychosis, and menopausal exacerbation. Women are twenty to thirty times more likely to be hospitalized for a psychotic episode in the first month after delivery than at any other time in their life (Twomey, 2009), suggesting a connection to birthing and the transition to motherhood.

This book seeks to build a bridge between personal experiences, clinical insights, and critical theory by exploring the issue of women and psychosis from a variety of perspectives, including the sociological, psychological, historical, biological, theological, psychoanalytic, and literary. At the forefront of the book are first-person accounts intended to cultivate an interchange between theory and life. In the spirit of Open Dialogue, *Women & Psychosis* has a commitment to what Bakhtin describes as "polyphony," or the "co-existence of multiple, separate, and equally valid 'voices' or points of view" (Olson, Seikkula, & Ziedonis, 2014, p. 5). There are many ways of understanding the topic of women and psychosis—it is hoped that this book will foster dialogue between them.

REFERENCES

Chesler, P. (1972). *Women and madness*. New York: St. Martin's Griffin.
Davoine, F. & Gaudilliere, J. (2004). *History beyond trauma.* New York: Other Press.
Goffman, E. (1963). *Stigma: Notes on a management of spoiled identity*. London: Penguin Books.
Morgan, V. A., Castle, D. J., & Jablensky, A. V. (2008). Do women express and experience psychosis differently from men? Epidemiological evidence from the Australian National Study of Low Prevalence (Psychotic) Disorders. *Australian & New Zealand Journal of Psychiatry*, *42*(1), 74-82.
Olson, M., Seikkula, J. & Ziedonis, D. (2014). *The key elements of dialogic practice in Open Dialogue*. Worcester: The University of Massachusetts Medical School.
Rector, N. A. & Seeman, M. V. (1992). Auditory hallucinations in women and men. *Schizophrenia Research, 7*(3), 233-236. doi: 10.1016/0920-9964(92)90017-Y.
Seeman, M.V. (2012). Women and psychosis. *Womens Health (Lond), 8*(2), 215–224. doi: 10.2217/whe.11.97.
Twomey, T. M. (2009). *Understanding postpartum psychosis: A temporary madness*. Santa Barbara, CA: Praeger.
Ussher, J. (1992). *Women's madness: Misogyny or mental illness?* Amherst: University of Massachusetts Press.

NOTE

1. While writing this introduction, I became curious about the style of dress I was wearing during my experience in the CPEP. I have learned that the cheongsam is a symbol of gender equality. It is closely associated with ending the practice of foot-binding and the start of the women's liberation movement.

Introduction

Marie Brown and Marilyn Charles

Women and Psychosis: Multidisciplinary Perspectives is a book that seeks to understand the interplay of two marginalized identities, those deemed "psychotic" and women. Although there have been many books on the broader topic of "women and madness," what makes this volume unique is its interdisciplinary approach, both in content and in form. The book is divided into four main sections: *Women & Psychosis in Arts & Culture*; *Women, Psychosis & the Body*; *Women, Psychosis & Spirituality*; and *Psychiatric Perspectives on Women & Psychosis*. Each of these sections reflects the varied, overarching discourses that surround the topic of women and psychosis. Within each section, we have attempted to include various forms of epistemology. For example, some chapters are theoretical, whereas others are scientific, first-person, or historical, and some chapters are a blend of several of these. In creating this collection, we found it imperative that all forms of knowing be considered in their own right, especially with regard to first-person accounts. Too often, people deemed "mad," particularly women, have had their experiences colonized or explained by others, whether by theory or by science. What constitutes "knowledge" or "truth" is dictated by those with institutional power, historically foreclosed to both women and those considered "mad." When women's "madness narratives" do appear in academic books, they are often positioned as primary sources to be analyzed and dissected by academic discourse and not as forms of knowledge in their own right. Therefore, in drawing both from feminism and Mad Studies, we included these narratives side-by-side with more institutional or "established" forms of knowing (e.g., psychiatric, theoretical). Our intent here is to intentionally disrupt traditional academic texts in a way that honors marginalized women's subjective experiences of what is commonly called "psychosis."

PART ONE: WOMEN & PSYCHOSIS IN ARTS & CULTURE

The chapters that comprise this section comment on the theme of women and psychosis through social and creative contexts. Although quite distinct in their approach, these four chapters each grapple with the following questions: what are the unique social, political, and personal contexts that bring women to experience "madness"? How can "madness" be a teacher? What gifts or insights can it bring to the experiencer, her family, and her social world? In reflecting on these questions, each chapter brings out the importance of story and story-telling.

Charles focuses on the relationship between social context and the manifestation of madness in women. In doing so, she traverses across several terrains, including the visual arts, literature, and psychotherapy. In particular, Charles illuminates the way in which women are often subordinate to the creative strivings of others, pushed into diminished social roles. Through the psychodynamic lens of a practicing clinician, Charles lends insight into the ways in which psychotherapeutic practice can help women locate themselves within familial and socio-political narratives. Both within art and within the therapy space, Charles stresses the importance of story-telling and of "writing" one's own narrative. She states,

> [. . .] stories help us to encounter social conventions from a new perspective, offering the possibility of a new reading of ideas and of catching glimpses of truths that may be hiding in plain sight, truths we might intuit without being able to articulate or that have become so accepted within the social fabric that they are not easily questioned.

Charles concludes that in working with story, what is often seen as "mad" can be understood as a meaningful response to a particular context as well as a means of exploring what she calls, "the complexities of existence."

Helen DeVinney's chapter focuses more literally on story, providing a comprehensive meditation on the literary trope of the madwoman. Most importantly, DeVinney takes an intersectional stance toward interpreting this figure, seeking to understand her within the context of multiple politics of identity. DeVinney takes us through prior feminist understandings of the literary madwoman (such as Gilbert and Gubar's classic text *The Madwoman in the Attic*) before developing her more third-wave approach. Rather than fall toward global notion regarding who the madwoman represents, DeVinney focuses on why she appears in the first place, asking the question: what is the greater purpose of her repeated appearances in literature? Using the theoretical contributions of R. D. Laing, Northrop Frye, and Rebecca Solnit, DeVinney speaks of the madwoman's call for us to "bear witness to her truth" and bring her into contact with our own personal narratives. She states,

A reader does not need to explain the madwoman's purpose or actions, she needs to recognize her story, direct others to her story, and perhaps, relate to the madwoman's story. In this recognition and sharing of personal narrative, the past is integrated instead of compartmentalized, a dialogue is created, and the false-self system is dismantled both at the level of the individual and at the level of society.

The third chapter, by Berta Britz, is personal contribution which she titles, most appropriately, "Stories." Britz's personal narrative of trauma and anomalous experiences speaks to the way in which imposed narratives by others led her to experience limiting beliefs about herself. Her story is a deeply personal and moving testament to the true power of story and story-telling. She states,

I will use stories to highlight the impact of gender, culture, and context across generations. They are stories about my relationship to "the other," stories about the meaning I made of "the other" in me, in family and in culture, and the meaning I made of "the other" outside me. They are stories of movement from a binary vision of myself and others that reflected dominant family/societal/cultural presuppositions about ethics, health, disease, gender, sex roles, sexual orientations, politics and power, to a dynamic and inclusive acceptance of self and co-creation of self in relation to "other" from a "both/and" perspective.

Together, these three chapters synergistically help to re-write the dominant narrative surrounding women and "psychosis," recognizing this phenomenon as deeply personal as well as socio-political.

PART TWO: WOMEN, PSYCHOSIS & THE BODY

In this section, we consider ways in which psychosis can result when women's relationships with their bodies are undermined or misunderstood. In her chapter, "Snakes in the Crib: Psychosocial Factors in Postpartum Psychosis," Marie Brown raises the important and neglected subject of postpartum psychosis. She first highlights that neglect itself as a meaningful marker of the tendency to pathologize the female body. Notably, marks Brown, postpartum psychosis is not even recognized as a problem in its own right but rather is inserted as a modifier to other disorders without sufficient recognition of the contextual nature of the disturbance. In contrast to that position, Brown stresses the importance of listening to the voice of lived experience. She notes that the tendency to sensationalize impedes understanding of the larger sociocultural issues.

Brown notes the remarkable dearth of nonmedical treatments and the lack of research and scholarship on psychological treatments in this area. Lack of valuing of women and their experience has led to pressures toward protecting the child at the expense of the mother and trends toward "quick fixes" that often do more harm than good, such as electroconvulsive therapy, which can often be more punitive than helpful. Such cultural devaluation also leads to psychological sequelae, such as guilt and a sense of loss of control. Other consequences include problems with partners and fears regarding future pregnancies. Opposing these trends, Brown stresses that social support aids recovery for women who have suffered from postpartum psychotic experiences.

In her chapter, "Disordered Eating and Disordered Thinking in Women: A Continuum in Objectification in Anorexia and Psychosis," Jessica Arenella highlights the ways in which sociocultural forces create risk factors in young women. Ideas of the body as primarily important in its visual appeal rather than it functions, health, or vitality promote unhealthy dieting, weight loss, and disordered eating. In this way, ideas associated with eating disorders can be seen as risk factors or preliminary stages of psychotic disturbance. Arenella notes that what has been termed the *anorexic voice* is similar to the voices encountered in psychosis, each linked to abuse histories and to ambivalence regarding the female role. Socially and interpersonally induced shame in relation to need compounds the difficulties and makes it even more difficult to adaptively fill those needs. Arenella also notes ways in which there can be a collision between sexual desire and prohibitions against such desires.

Following Arieti, Arenella views disordered eating as a narrowing of focus in relation to intolerable anxiety. Because this narrowing of focus tends to preclude resolution of the underlying problem, the "solution" becomes addictive. Given that part of the underlying problem has to do with unattainable cultural demands regarding the body, young women who are at risk for developing disordered eating or psychosis, and whose internal resources are insufficient to meet developmental demands, need assistance in facing such challenges, including recognition that there are external obstacles to be faced; that the fault does not lie entirely within. From that frame of reference, contends Arenella, those who are suffering from eating disorders and psychosis put "into sharp relief, at much detriment to themselves, the pathology of our culture and time."

PART THREE: WOMEN, PSYCHOSIS & SPIRITUALITY

This section focuses on ways in which psychosis may at times represent a misreading of women's experience. In her chapter, "Mystics, Witches, or Hysterics? The Therapeutic Stakes when Spirituality Becomes Symptom," Liane Carlson offers us the story of Geneviève L., a woman who was taken to be mad in the late nineteenth century in Europe. Paradoxically, this "mad" woman was seeking a woman of her time who was taken to be, not mad, but rather inspired. Through this lens, Carlson considers the relationship between the madwoman and the sage, the madwoman and the saint, and, by extension, the relationship between psychosis, religion, and hysteria. Notably, she contends such distinctions depend on the frame of reference that configures the lens through which the question is considered. Carlson posits the diagnosis of psychosis as a value judgement that overrides and denies the value of subjective truths. Early descriptors of symptoms, she notes, explicitly focused solely on medical observations with no interest in what the person herself might report. At the time being considered, the Church was concerned with the medical potential for deriding sainthood. Their credibility was at stake.

The question of the legitimacy of the woman's mind and meaning, Carlson argues, is what led these various debates to circle around hysteria as a biological vulnerability *in need of male interpretation.* The emphasis on photography fixed the visual as symptom display, leaving the emphasis in hysteria on signs over content. In the controversy between medical and religious interpretations, there was a tension between the offering by religion to make the suffering sufferable versus the medical view that proposed that the problem was biological. Using hysteria as a frame of reference, the symptoms could be seen as potentially both religious and erotic. Alternatively, the feminist view insists that meanings and symptoms are socially constructed. From that frame of reference, the turn toward religion for Geneviève L. might be seen as both a rebellion and an escape in a time of limited possibilities.

In her chapter, "From Sick to Gifted: Discovering Shamanic Illness," Gogo Ekhaya Esima extends the theme of postpartum vulnerabilities from a personal perspective. Therapy, for her, was not helpful and did not provide a sense of being understood, and medications just clouded her mind and feelings. Treatment merely continued the cycle of lack of respect for the individual by those claiming to be responsible. Medications, in particular, were a source of disconnection, not only from her feelings and creative energies but also from her children. Without social support, her gifts and talents were taxing and hard to sustain or make use of.

For Esima, the recovery movement provides an important basis of social support through which to live one's life rather than to mobilize an identity as a mental patient. In this way, she takes a stand for the importance of being able to obtain resources through which to live one's life as it comes, and learning to tolerate difficulties and make use of one's capacities. Notably, it was the spiritual path that helped Esima to face trauma rather than be destroyed by it, assisted by others who had made that journey. In this way, the primary lesson offered is the importance of respectful engagement with those who are struggling so as to provide maximum support for them in their own journeys.

PART FOUR: PSYCHIATRIC PERSPECTIVES ON WOMEN & PSYCHOSIS

In the final section of the book, we present two chapters on women and psychosis from a psychiatric perspective. First is the contribution of Simone Ciufolini and Nicola Byrne, two psychiatrists working in the United Kingdom. In their chapter, these authors synthesize the theoretical and clinical literature on psychosis with the everyday, through the use of case studies. Beginning with an understanding of how psychiatry understands psychosis, they then go on to discuss how psychosis from a bio-medical perspective is distinct between men and women, including treatment considerations. For example, the authors discuss how antipsychotic medications may be particularly concerning for women due to their potential to compromise fertility and increase osteoporosis. The authors also make distinctions between various diagnoses across the psychosis spectrum, advocating for reduced medical interventions in the case of psychological (i.e., trauma-related) psychotic symptoms, such as those in borderline personality disorder. The authors also describe the current literature related to psychosis and trauma more broadly with a focus on gender differences. They then cover hormonal and neurological differences in women as they may impact the course of psychosis and treatment. Lastly, Ciufolini and Bryne present these research findings through the lens of three different composite case studies of women they have worked with in the NHS in South London. Each case presents various ways in which these psychiatrists have tailored treatments to fit the unique psychosocial factors of each woman.

Mary Seeman, a Canadian psychiatrist, then provides a focus specifically on the construct of schizophrenia and the way in which this diagnosis is expressed differently in men and women. Her contribution is an extensive search of the biopsychosocial literature from 1990–2016. Her chapter describes the ways in which women diagnosed with schizophrenia have an advantage over their male counterparts, in terms of social, economic, and psychiatric outcomes. She, however, cautions that women diagnosed with schizophrenia often have added complications related to traditional gender roles including care-taking and maternal responsibilities, and that these factors are often neglected in psychiatric treatment. Seeman also describes premorbid risk factors as they relate to the brain and body, presenting differences in trauma, risk-taking, and substance use in men and women as they relate to the manifestation of illness. Taken together, these two chapters are representative of a psychiatric perspective on the topic of women and psychosis, offering insight into the ways in which the physical body is thought to play a role. This final section rounds out the themes being considered in this volume, to include the psychiatric contexts in which ideas of madness are constructed along with the sociocultural, embodied, spiritual, and experiential aspects.

I

WOMEN & PSYCHOSIS IN ARTS & CULTURE

Chapter One

Women and Madness in Context

Marilyn Charles

Prejudice, intolerance, and stigma are so intrinsically part of the social fabric that they can become relatively invisible. The gendering of social roles in ways that undermine women's development results in what LaCapra (1999) refers to as a *structural trauma* that can invite a strident reactivity or a masochistic surrender in relation to oppressive social forces that become internalized in ways that invite self-hatred and feelings of inferiority (Pheterson, 1990). Women in western culture have become caught up in a forced binary, in which the extant power structures have devalued basic human values such as empathy in favor of "objective," rational knowledge (Gilligan & Richards, 2009) in ways that undermine the ability to recognize and respond to the signal functions of affect so crucial to psychosocial development. Reading women's emotionality as a problem, without trying to understand the contexts in which the symptoms have arisen, tends to amplify the distress, at times driving them toward psychosis (Charles & O'Loughlin, 2013).

Oppressive social forces invite shame in the individual, making it difficult to fight the oppression (Charles, 2011). Recognizing internalized oppression as an *appropriated* oppression contextualizes individual difficulties within the sociocultural contexts that give rise to them (Tappan, 2006). Because mastery and ownership are important aspects of identity development, to the extent that the woman is invited into an identity that denies fundamental aspects of her being, she is both devalued and diminished (Tappan, 2005). That appropriated oppression, if unrecognized and unexplored, is then passed along from mother to daughter through the dialogical process of identity formation, seen both in the sociocultural discourse (Bakhtin, 1981) and also in studies that link identity development to evolving narratives between parent and child (Fivush et al., 2011). Their subordinate status in western culture has resulted in women being defined in relation to that status, impeding the woman's ability to articulate her own values or to define herself in her own terms (Miller, 1976). Liberation from entrenched sociocultural oppression requires first recognizing ways in which prevailing myths and images are oppressive so that we can develop new, more empowering stories (Tappan, 2005). At the sociocultural level, the psychoanalytic lens affords insights into the problems in ways that might invite effective and adaptive change. At the individual level, the psychoanalytic lens provides a means for recognition and exploration through which the woman might break the cycle of intergenerational transmission of internalized oppression, find and claim her own voice, and authorize her own becoming.

In a world in which history has been written primarily by men, the woman's voice has been muted and her place has often been that of the silent shadow, standing to the side and not speaking directly. This legacy leaves her in a somewhat "sinister" position, relieving when she can be kept in her place but unnerving when she insists on taking a more direct stand. Although the feminist movement has raised our awareness of some of the difficulties inherent in this gendering of power and knowledge, many of the resulting problems remain invisible, thus allowing them to persist. That persistence has resulted in confusion for many women between the personal and societal dimensions of traumatic experience (Charles, 2011) and over the value of human relationship versus commodification in western industrialized societies (Layton, 2004). Perhaps most fundamentally, powerlessness has left women angry over injustice, but gender socialization has impeded women's ability to make use of their anger in constructive ways, particularly in patriarchal cultures (Thomas, 2005).

Historically, attributions of *madness* often index ideas or behavior that are inconvenient, offensive, or not easy to understand. And yet, as Hornstein (2009) notes, *"madness is more code than chemistry,"* (p. xix; italics in original), impossible to understand outside of the context through which the code might be recognized. Madness, as one form of human experience and behavior, can only be understood within the personal, familial, and sociocultural and historical contexts that give rise to it. From that perspective, the extent to which we value the individual voice and attempt to understand the contexts within which that voice makes sense links back to an ethical stand regarding the value of the individual and her experience.

In this chapter, I will be examining madness in relation to difficulties facing women in western society, as industrialization has afforded both greater opportunities and also more intense pressures toward subordination and commodification. The appearance of respect or *equal opportunity* in western cultures can make it difficult to recognize tensions between whatever women might uniquely contribute to the world versus societal demands to maintain relationships. Cultural forces that push them toward relational values over autonomy have made it difficult for women to realize their own creative potential, often resolving these tensions by fostering their partners' creative efforts rather than their own. Opposing such societal constraints, many female artists have struggled to assert their own individuality in relation to the work of their partners, at times ravaged by the lack of recognition of their own unique talents and value (Ayral-Clause, 2002). As Lee Krasner puts it: "I'm always going to be Mrs. Jackson Pollock—that's a matter of fact—[but] I painted before Pollock, during Pollock, after Pollock" (2016).

I will describe some of the ways in which women have been driven *mad* by cultural forces that have silenced and constrained them. I use this term advisedly, to register the relationship between the power structures that both deny women resources and also suppress their legitimate anger, thereby turning anger mad/anger into mad/despair and distress (Thomas, 2005). Examples will be offered of creative women for whom cultural values literally have displaced their power and autonomy by rendering them "mad" in ways that obstructed their development. Ironically, it may be their creativity that pushes some women up against the very forces that serve to oppress them. I will first look through the lens of culture to describe ways in which difference has been problematic for the woman such that her very creativity may become a hazard. I will then describe the clinical context, through which we are afforded insight into the particular ways in which devaluation can pass along the generations, impeding mothers' abilities to offer their daughters a secure base (Charles et al., 2001), and also ways in which the consulting room can offer a space within which the individual can locate herself within the narrative as it has developed and find her own voice.

THE SOCIOCULTURAL CONTEXT

For centuries, physicians have attempted to better understand ways in which sociocultural factors are implicated in women's madness (Busfield, 1988; Hirschbein, 2010). Freud, then, further complicated this research by delving into the psyches of women but always in relation to the standard of male development (Breuer & Freud, 1893–1895). The depiction of women as objects rather than subjects has continued, as noted by feminists and cultural theorists (de Lauretis, 1984; Walker, 1994). This objectification complicates their coming-into-being as individual subjects. Depictions of women in the media are often caricatures that, although we may reject them consciously, still leave a stain, a point of darkness that colors our vision without itself being visible. The cinema, in particular, has become a powerful purveyor of cultural meanings, including the familiar trope of woman as excess, the woman as mad (Charles, 2004).

Our discomfort with difference has too often resulted in rendering the woman as mad, a theme explored very directly in documentaries such as Light's (1993) *Dialogues with Madwomen* and Collins' (2000) *We Don't Live Under Normal Conditions.* Such documentaries enable women to speak for themselves about ways in which "treatment" can be used in oppressive and retaliatory ways, affirming the importance of safeguarding the woman's right to define her own needs and desires. These explorations also highlight the importance of turning our lenses back on our own culture, so that we might see ourselves from another angle that allows us to question whatever might otherwise be hiding in plain sight. As de Lauretis (1984) puts it: experience "is produced not by external ideas, values, or material causes, but by one's personal, subjective, engagement in the practices, discourses, and institutions that lend significance (value, meaning, and affect) to the events of the world" (p. 159).

Truth often hides behind the very tropes that become so commonplace that we fail to question them. The theme of the madwoman has become a familiar trope in literature as well, highlighting the fear and allure of madness, and the ways in which that tension can be projected into the woman as a symbol of projected dread (Van Buren, 1994). From a psychoanalytic perspective, the frightening madwoman—the witch who threatens to devour and destroy—may be seen as a displacement of the terror of engulfment in relation to the desire and fear of being re-absorbed into the all-powerful early mother. Early symbiotic entanglements with mother leave us caught in a developmental trajectory in which the desire for transformation is in some ways inextricable from the dread of loss and annihilation (Klein, 1975). The more intense the emotion, the more difficult it can be to disentangle internal oppression from external, leaving us oppressed by an external force that cannot be fought directly because of its illusory nature. Moderating the anxiety, then, can only truly be accomplished if we can recognize the internal fears in relation to the developmental demands. Too often, however, we develop elaborate defenses that become compelling rationales for sustaining the status quo. Even well-intentioned systems of "care," such as medical diagnosis and treatment, can sometimes become mechanisms for oppression and constraint to the extent that the people who are treated are not met with sufficient respect for their own individual perspectives and desires (Hornstein, 2009).

Such disrespect is dangerous because it impedes identity development, thereby increasing the risk of later destabilization (Charles, 2011, 2014a; Dimen, 2003). Early fears are compelling, in part because they become embedded in the body in ways that make it difficult to even consciously recognize them, much less work them through. The fear of engulfment by the early mother can keep us caught between the desire for growth and evasive actions that move in precisely the opposite direction. Affective intensity can immobilize us, impeding our ability to follow our own path in spite of our fears, to surrender to possibility in ways that might be transformative (Ghent, 1990). Such surrender can only be viable to the extent that internal resources and external support provide sufficient safety.

Not only women but also men are impacted by ideas about human development that deprecate more implicit and less conscious ways of making sense of experience (Belenky et al., 1986). Dichotomization of mind and body impedes the integration of sensory and rational data so essential for healthy development (Charles, 2011). For the man, whose identity has been built on distinguishing and disentangling himself from the mother, fear of engulfment may be particularly problematic, leaving him out of touch with the very affective signals through which we make sense of self and experience (Diamond, 2004). Displacing that fear onto women provides a means for distancing from it but, as with all projections, there is always the threat of return. Paradoxically, then, it is precisely what is displaced and disavowed that looms largest, but now as an *external* rather than an *internal* threat. Managing the problem posed by women, then, has often been done in ways that diminish her and her threat, and also mark her as inferior and incapable. Social change increases threat, also exacerbating discriminatory practices (Morton et al., 2009). From that perspective, taking on the role of protector is a viable solution for the man who can find a woman who is willing to take on the complementary role of victim/protectee, and who also becomes responsible for carrying and managing emotions.

To the extent that the protector role is overly constraining or demanding, the needs of the woman become inconvenient and even threatening. It is in this context that the "protected" status of woman as property becomes highly dangerous to her being and becoming. In western culture, the very male figure who served as protector, historically, also had the authority to judge the woman under his protection as "mad" if she failed to fulfill her expected social role. The French sculptor Camille Claudel, for example, managed to survive a period of great distress under the protective support of her father. A week after his death, however, she was sent to an asylum by her brother, where she remained institutionalized until her death thirty years later (Paris, 1998). Elizabeth Packard was more fortunate. Although she was committed to an asylum for three years in the 1860s by her husband because of her insistence on maintaining her own religious and ethical views, she was able to effectively advocate for her release. Subsequently, she fought to protect the rights of women and to change commitment laws, safeguarding the individual's right to a hearing to determine sanity (Carlisle, 2010).

As voices were increasingly raised against the abuses being perpetrated as a function of these social inequities in western culture, the plight of the creative—and inconvenient—woman became increasingly visible. Powerful voices in France and England at the end of the eighteenth century paved the way for nineteenth century debates regarding how women might be freed from the subordination inherent in the family as it had existed (Hutcheson, 1983). In the later nineteenth and early twentieth centuries, as women were becoming more active in advocating for their own views and desires, tensions mounted between personal and social definitions of possibilities for women, claims for individual freedom versus demands of the extant social order (Hutcheson, 1983).

THE LITERARY CONTEXT

Given the limited power of women in that era, literature became one means for authors and readers to explore some of these social and cultural constraints. And yet, even the literature of that time that marks women's desires for independence, in the context of restrictive ideas about femininity and the ostensible place of the woman, contains characters who are often "forced into contrived and essentially false reconciliations of sense and sensibility" (Hutcheson, 1989, p. 238). Late nineteenth-century writers such as George Eliot, who explored through her novels ways in which circumscribed gender roles impeded development for both men and women, seemed to be ultimately constrained by social demands that led toward self-abnegation and restraint, submission rather than self-fulfillment, a favored resolution to the problem of female desire in that era (Machann, 2005). Eliot likely, however, paved the way for later writers such as Virginia Woolf (1928, 1929), who pushed up against the edges of societal constraints quite explicitly in her writings, as she struggled in her own life between conventionality and the creative strivings that at times seemed to pull her toward madness (see, for example, Charles 2015).

Literature is a powerful tool for such considerations because it invites the reader to explore various possibilities, through an engagement with a text that can feel quite real. As George Eliot puts it: "Art is the nearest thing to life; it is a mode of amplifying experience and extending contact with our fellow-men beyond the bounds of our personal lot" (1963, p. 83). Our readings are guided by the author who focuses our gaze, providing the type of vicarious experience that Gallese (2009) terms *embodied simulation*, in which we try an experience or a way of being on for size. The reader is invited into an affective engagement that can simulate a social interaction, including the affective tone and coloration that lends richness to the experience (Mar & Oatley, 2008; Miall & Kuiken, 1994). In that way, stories help us to encounter social conventions from a new perspective, offering the possibility of a new reading of ideas and of catching glimpses of truths that may be hiding in plain sight, truths we might intuit without being able to articulate or that have become so accepted within the social fabric that they are not easily questioned. Literature provides a useful potential space because it can be familiar without necessarily being personal; it is both about us and not-us. As the story develops, the reader can begin to see how meanings increasingly formulate around signs that become symbols as we gain greater facility in reading them. In this way, women's stories have provided opportunities for readers to move beyond conventional meanings of distress and madness, so that they might grapple with the social injustice often hidden within the narrative (Hornstein, 2009).

Literary devices, such as metonymy and metaphor, condense meanings in ways that pull the reader into the more experiential, affective aspects of knowing. Metaphors afford a bit of distance, the safety of a transitional space through which we can play with ideas and face difficult or inconvenient truths. But the images attendant to these metaphors are linked to emotions that organize meanings (Bucci, 2001) and also invite a concrete and embodied engagement with the text. As feelings intensify, our kinesthetic responsiveness to the structure, rhythms, and other formal aspects of the text are heightened (Jackson, Meltzoff, & Decety, 2006; Kilintari et al., 2016), allowing what Forrest (1969) calls "the kinesthetic sensuousness of literature" (p. 457), through which reason may be bypassed, as emotional responsiveness conveys a sense of "truth" in the experience.

At the other extreme, however, literature also can invite reflection through the coexistence and layering of meanings and possibilities. Fiction affords a means for keeping our balance as we engage in possibilities that may seem alien, through a displacement that allows us to keep one foot on the solid ground of our own experience. In this way, the reader can both identify and dis-identify with characters and dilemmas as they are encountered within the text. The distance afforded by the displacement helps to moderate our defenses, opposing the tendency to *turn a blind eye* (Bion, 1977) to difficult meanings, so that a scene or memory might be constituted in a way that allows us to find our way into a story that resists being told. In this way, literature provides a useful means for social comment and exploration.

At times, our gaze may be focused in ways that elude or even oppose our conscious values or intentions. The hazard of the well-told story is that we might fail to notice as we become caught up in problematic or even potentially destructive renderings of the human experience. One may read *Jane Eyre*, for example, utterly caught up in the perspective of the narrator, for whom the madwoman in the attic is presented as inhuman. "In the deep shade, whether it was beast or human being, one figure ran backwards and forwards. What it was, whether beast or human being, one could not, at first sight, tell; it grovelled, seemingly, on all fours; it snatched and growled like some strange wild animal; but it was covered with clothing, and a quantity of dark, grizzled hair, wild as a mane, hid its head and face" (Brontë, 2006, p. 212).

Rochester dubs his wife a lunatic, thereby denying her humanity. In so doing, he justifies in his own mind her displacement that allows him to wed the woman of his choice with impunity, "this young girl who stands so grave and quiet at the mouth of hell, looking collectedly at the gambols of a demon" (p. 213). Jane Eyre, however, cannot deny the reality of the bond between these two human beings and must leave the man she loves lest she be further enchanted by *his* madness, exemplified in his denial of the humanity of the other.

In reading *Jane Eyre,* it is easy to become so caught up in the dilemma of the two lovers that one accepts the designation of the madwoman in the attic as beast and lunatic, unhuman and inconvenient. Our position may be invisible to us as a perspective—rather than a reality—until we are confronted with an alternate view. It is startling, then, to experience this disjunction in *Wide Sargasso Sea,* where we encounter Jean Rhys's (1966) re-rendering of this same character, this madwoman in the attic. This time, however, we are offered a biographical sketch of Antoinette Mason as a person in her own right. Rhys, in re-writing Antoinette in the first person, from her own perspective, enables us to recognize the clash that occurs when Antoinette encounters Rochester and the two find themselves tied together in ways that become terrible and deadly for each.

Rhys offers us a rendering that highlights ways in which culture and context can drive a person beyond their limits, rendering them mad/insane to the extent that their madness/anger has no power to affect their circumstance. In this sense, both Antoinette (dubbed "Bertha" by Rochester) and Rochester are driven mad by their union but each feels powerless to end that union. Antoinette hopes to force love but only incurs further hatred by the man who feels imprisoned by her. Rochester, in turn, tries to force Antoinette to become the "Bertha" he might love but only invites further alienation through this denial—and hatred—of her actual personhood. In this portrayal, we are able to see how strikingly reality can clash with illusion and how dangerous a power imbalance can be in such circumstances. Not only does Rochester's dominion over Antoinette destroy her, it also proves highly destructive to him and to those he loves.

In *Jane Eyre,* the author turns this truth on its head, inviting the reader to accept as positive and legitimate the happy ending that is achieved through the sacrifice of the madwoman in the attic. In Jean Rhys's account, however, that same ending is rendered as a release from hell, from imprisonment by the man who has controlled Antoinette's life and even meaning itself. This dilemma, in which a woman's well-being, freedom, and even her very life could be held in the hands of the man seen by society as accountable for her, has been longstanding in Western society, where women historically have been rendered as property rather than beings in their own right (Edwards, 2011; Murphy, 2013).

CONTEXTUALIZING MADNESS

This is the dilemma highlighted in Geller and Harris's (1994) *Women of the Asylum*, showing how women historically have been imprisoned against their will, often by male family members, for behavior or views deemed aberrant or deviant from the extant societal norms. From this vantage point, one can see ways in which societal standards and psychiatric diagnoses could read the woman as mad, and then the conditions of confinement could truly drive her mad. This fact—that one can, indeed, be driven mad, is at the core of current research that shows ways in which psychosis is a function of trauma, such that the conditions that may have driven a person mad must always be our first consideration (see, for example, Hammersley, Read, Woodall & Dillon, 2007; Longden & Read, 2016). These data demand that we look first at the contexts in which symptoms have arisen rather than merely ascribing the source of difference or deviation to the person's character or physiology. That sociocultural perspective is in direct opposition to the current trend toward a medicalization of distress and categorization of symptoms into diagnostic categories that are meant to facilitate treatment but which may add further burdens without ameliorating distress. When the causes of distress are environmental, focusing treatment at the level of character or symptom tends to merely blur communications that, as noted previously, represent attempts to speak to underlying problems for which there have been no words. The failure to recognize contextual factors can render such communications of distress meaningless and therefore mad (see, for example, Charles & O'Loughlin, 2013).

Women of the Asylum followed Chesler's (1972) ground-breaking *Women and Madness,* which shows how patriarchy has shaped societal definitions of sanity and madness, and also how psychiatry can serve as a weapon of social control. Chesler describes how psychiatric diagnosis has targeted deviations from sex-role stereotypes and labeled these deviations as "mad," thereby constraining and pathologizing individual choice. Recognizing ways in which labels can obscure and enforce meanings has helped to further enquiries into ways in which class and race also affect diagnosis, treatment and the likelihood of becoming marginalized by psychiatric diagnoses and injunctions (see, for example, Netjek, Allison & Hilburn, 2012).

Increasingly, there is recognition that social inequalities interact with one another in ways that change over time, requiring ongoing study of psychotic experience as it emerges in and is reported by women (Woodman & Wyn, 2015). Ample evidence affirms that much of what we term "mental illness" can only be understood in relation to the socio-cultural contexts in which it has arisen, and that interventions that acknowledge and address the contextual nature of distress are most effective (Charles & O'Loughlin, 2013). For example, in Northern Finland, teams of health workers respond to a first psychotic break by going into the family home and discussing with the family the problems that family members are experiencing (Seikkula & Olson, 2003). This type of intervention—that actively invites reflective function in family members—has resulted in a drastic reduction of chronicity in psychotic illness. (Reflective function refers to the capacity to mentalize, to have ideas about how one functions as a thinking, feeling being in relation to others who have their own perspectives as well.) Further, evidence shows that marginalization itself exacerbates distress such that attending to the person's links to family and community are an important aspect of any healing or recovery process (Charles, 2013; Lynam & Cowley, 2007). From that perspective, if we wish to transform the causes of suffering rather than merely deaden the distress signals, we must recognize ways in which cultural structures and practices obstruct development and increase suffering, and address the larger social contexts in which symptoms have emerged.

Complicating these issues are familial factors, such as the intergenerational transmission of mourning, that can interfere with the parental attunement so integral to healthy self-development (Charles, 2014b; van Ijzendoorn, Schuengel, & Bakermans-Kranenburg, 1999). When it is difficult for the parent to hold the child in mind, it is difficult for the child to hold herself in mind and thereby to develop a solid, stable, and resilient identity structure. That instability impedes the ability to be adaptive and resilient in the face of further stressors, heightening the risk of later severe psychological disturbance (Hammersley, Read, Woodall, & Dillon, 2007) and, at the extreme, driving children toward dissociation and other symptoms of psychosis (Liotti, 2004).

Cultural devaluation invites shame, which impedes social interaction and inhibits curiosity (Tomkins, 1982), making it difficult to take the types of risks required for new learning and the experiences of mastery that build positive self-regard and help to develop the metacognitive capacities so crucial to reflective function (Fonagy, Gergely, Jurist, & Target, 2002, Lysaker et.al., 2011). Because identity is built in the context of relationships, the mother who cannot sufficiently value herself as a woman communicates that devaluation to her daughter (Main & Hesse, 1990). For girls growing up in families in which females are devalued, it is difficult to build a secure and valued sense of self. Insufficient grounding in a stable and coherent identity leaves fault lines in the self that result in greater vulnerability to stress across the life cycle (Parkes, Stevensen-Hinde, & Maris, 1991). That is why attuned and attentive psychotherapy can be so important to assist those for whom this process has gone awry. Insight-oriented therapies that privilege the development of subjective understanding and voice may be particularly important for marginalized groups, including women, who need to be able to determine their own goals, values, and direction in a world that may be fundamentally at odds with that progression. Encountering someone who is able to stand separate from, but in respectful relation to, the person seeking assistance is crucial.

THE CLINICAL CONTEXT—WORKING OUTSIDE THE LINES

Although psychosis is often thought of in terms of internal deficits, even very bright and creative children can fall through the gaps left by parents who are not able to provide the type of attuned, respectful tracking so crucial to healthy development. At times, children need to be able to learn precisely what their parents cannot tell them, truths that have been lost behind layers of silence across the generations. To add further layers to this discussion, I will draw on my clinical work to help the reader recognize the importance of respectful engagement with those who have become lost in relation to themselves. Notably, I do believe that people are *driven* mad and therefore need to learn as much as possible about the contexts in which their symptoms occur. Such individuals need assistance in building affect tolerance and narrative coherence within the context of a relationship that is safe enough to be able to discover oneself as a unique individual in relation to another. That exploration helps to build a more solid identity structure, providing greater equilibrium, resilience and the possibility of choosing more adaptive living environments and means of coping.

Equilibrium depends on the ability to respond to internal signals effectively and adaptively. In families in which feelings are denied and denigrated, women often carry the affect but then suffer from disrespectful attitudes towards the very feelings that mark the problem (Charles, 2001). That disregard is compounded by "treatments" that blunt feelings and obscure affective signals rather than helping the person to make meaning from them. For example, as a young child, Ava[1] seemed to thrive within the safe containment of her loving parents, working happily on various creative enterprises. When she needed more than the parents could provide, however, her frustration resulted in angry outbursts that wounded the mother, who was invested in her identity as a "good" mother. When the mother became hurt and anxious, the father became protective and angry, and Ava was left further isolated within her distress, deepening her sense that some inchoate internal badness was at play in her.

The parents' inability to help her to recognize, name, and manage her conflicting emotions, and to work through the interpersonal conflicts within the family, left Ava utterly unprepared to build relationships in the outer world. Unable to build a solid foundation, she retreated further into fantasy, calling upon her creativity and intelligence to jump past difficulties rather than confronting them. Eventually, she was left utterly isolated and alone, unable to build relationships or even a substantial body of creative work.

With no coherent, stable sense of self from which to act, there was no path forward and no way to build anything that felt solid, real, reliable, or valuable, eventually resulting in psychotic symptoms and the fear that she was losing her mind.

Maternal failures to provide adequate holding and containment leave the daughter with no strong maternal model for identification. Too often, then, the resolution to the developmental impasse seems to be either to become *like* the father or to sufficiently please the man who will become the source of salvation. Such a move further estranges the young woman from herself as an active agent and the potential source of desire, satisfaction and creative engagement. Even otherwise capable young women can find themselves freezing in a moment when the needs of the other would seem to countermand their own, and self-abnegation seems to be the price of relationship.

Without a secure sense of identity, the young woman can find herself frighteningly seeming mad at the threshold to adulthood. No longer protected by whatever had been "home," attempts to make the transition to adulthood reveal the fault lines in self-development. Paradoxically, the inability to look at and work through problems can make the family something of a protective time bomb, such that leaving the nest activates the explosion. In such families, the identified patient is often the repository of the family secrets, told in coded form through the symptom.

These types of entrenched problems, when unresolved, continue to haunt future generations because of the failures that repeat themselves. In this way, unresolved, intergenerational trauma often speaks across the generations through disrupted life narratives and psychotic symptoms that mark whatever has become unspeakable within the family (Davoine & Gaudillière, 2004). Psychotic symptoms can capture in concrete terms the metaphors and family myths that affect family members without being overtly recognized. Unacknowledged and unresolved, traumatic truths haunt us, distorting and undermining development. Atkinson (2002) describes these *trauma trails* as song lines, evocative melodies whose echoes can haunt us until we heed their call. This type of haunting tends to occur with what LaCapra (1999) terms *generalized* or *structural* trauma that is inherited rather than experienced directly (Abraham, 1975). When the trail of memory has been broken, we are left with ghosts and phantoms that hold us in their grasp until we can more fully constitute them in our minds and make sense of the stories they tell (Abraham & Torok, 1994; Apprey, 1993; Kavanaugh, 2012). That type of inchoate, historical, structural trauma is often internalized as an ineffable *absence* (LaCapra) or emptiness (Charles, 2000) that resists mourning, at times leaving symptoms that may be borne as stigmata that are unresolvable or even perversely gratifying. Making peace with unresolved pain can carry a high price.

Because of the essential unresolvability at its core, structural, generalized trauma can be experienced as a shameful, humiliating legacy that is difficult to repair. In Abraham's formulation, it is "the dead who were shamed during their lifetime or who took unspeakable secrets to the grave" who are most likely to haunt us (1975, p. 171). The denigration of women has left one such trauma trail, infused by the shame that is evoked by marginalization and abjection, and resists being worked through because it is so difficult to face. And so, the very family member who is most sensitive to the underlying disturbance, or who recognizes the point of vulnerability and sees that something important is at stake, can be warded off as a danger to the family system. When the family resists such knowledge, the bearer of the difficult truths may be attacked and driven crazy by the designation of craziness. Even today, young women may be driven mad because they stumble over inconvenient truths within the family and culture. To the extent that the culture affirms the family's version of reality, the person's hold on reality is further distended. Often, as with Ava, the child hits a limit within the family because one parent is protecting the other.

When the child needs more than the parent can provide, the parent's distress can invite the other parent to be angry at the child as the source of the distress. Ava became so derailed by this collusion of the parents that she was left with a sense of herself as inchoately but ultimately "bad," as though her needs were illegitimate and utterly unfillable. The legacy of this family dynamic was to thrust her unprepared into a world where she desperately sought solace but, in expecting none, managed to find none. There was no conceptual map through which to locate empathic concern as opposed to narcissistic entanglement. Her father's loving, affiliative self-absorption became the prototype for the beguiling, creative individuals she sought, who could recognize her gifts but not nurture her development.

When Ava originally entered my office at the Austen Riggs Center, she had come to a standstill at university, unable to make use of her high intelligence and creative potential, and fearful that she might be descending into madness. Her initial psychological assessment alarmed the evaluator, who said he had never seen such profound psychosis in a projective testing protocol. Because of my interest in trying to better understand the at-times fine line between creativity and madness, and ways in which creative women have been driven or rendered mad because of their difficulties in conforming to conventional social roles, I had explored links between creativity and psychosis in my research (Charles, Clemence & Biel, 2011; Charles, Durham-Fowler & Malone, 2016). I knew from this research that creative individuals, under strain, can become utterly ungrounded, resulting in disordered thinking that relieves when the distress is attenuated. That understanding helped me in my role as therapist to help the treatment team be less anxious about this young woman so that they could *hold* her anxiety rather than compounding it.

In this research, we had learned that vulnerability to disordered thinking could change over time in the course of intensive psychoanalytic therapy such that the person could find sufficient ground to maintain her creativity while also engaging in meaningful ways with others. In this way, psychoanalytic therapy can help women find the balance between idiosyncrasy and a grounding in consensual reality that affords the freedom required for creative endeavors. Notably, in our study, the poorest long-term outcomes were found, not with those whose responses seemed overtly psychotic, but with those whose resources were so strained that their responses were dull, banal, and overly controlled and constricted. These results make sense when you think about it, in that those who were too pressured by their symptoms to engage with the testing stimuli were likely also too pressured to make good use of therapeutic offerings. Too often, however, we do not think but rather merely react, and psychotic symptoms can be alarming. At Riggs, because we are working with dysregulation coming from many sides at all times, staff members recognize the importance of being able to downshift—to find a way to attenuate our own affect towards greater equilibrium—when *we* are losing our minds so that we might be able, once again, to actually think. Such experiences help us to confront the poignancy of the desire to medicate dysregulated individuals who dysregulate us, so that we can take on the more fundamental challenge of helping *them* to more effectively manage their *own* dysregulation so that they can make better use of their capacities in their lives.

Ava struggled with her desire to be creative against her fear of imminent collapse. Her psychiatrist suggested a trial of antipsychotics to forestall what the psychiatrist diagnosed as a tendency toward psychosis. In this country, low doses of antipsychotics are at times prescribed in this way. My own narrative, however, located Ava's symptoms within the context of development gone awry. Although it seemed to me that these stories were not incompatible, for Ava they were utterly at odds and she decided to stop working with her psychiatrist and place her trust in me. Thus began a difficult negotiation between her desire to instantaneously arrive at the place where she wanted to be and my sense that one must begin at the beginning, from wherever one is. The idea of learning has become oddly remote in this age in which facts are so massively accessible and less stress is place on the capacity to reflectively make use of them.

Ava had been unable to figure out how to bring her talents to bear in the world of her peers. An adored child of a limited mother and older father, neither parent had been able to help her learn to negotiate such challenges but rather encouraged her to override her experience in ways that left her further alienated from self and other. The father's death one year before had brought her out of the comfort of her illusory world. The fact of the loss afforded an edge that had been missing, a confrontation with reality that caught her attention but left her floundering.

Ava had been diagnosed with bipolar disorder in her early teens, and mood stabilizers provided sufficient relief that she remained convinced that this was the correct diagnosis. In college, she learned dialectical behavioral therapy as a way of further managing her distress. By the time I met her, her affect was so well managed that I found her difficult to engage with but rather often felt drowsy and unable to put together the threads of her story into a coherent narrative. Unable to concentrate, read, or write, Ava was certain that something was terribly wrong with her mind. Our work entailed us bumping into one another repeatedly. Her desire to by-pass the process of self-development, so that she might build an identity that might be pleasing to others, was met by my presumption that there was no way to build a life without looking inside and locating one's thoughts, feelings, values, and beliefs. Eventually, Ava resigned herself to the impossibility of building a self from without and began to face the pain within. That milestone marked the beginning of the very real work she has been doing in constructing a viable, resilient self, safeguarded by her increasing understanding of and empathy toward the distress she experiences in relation to the difficulties she encounters in her life. Her fear of madness has been replaced by fears of not being able to become all she longs to be. The latter is a challenge that can be faced, step by step, in the context of relationships in which she can be recognized.

Having a mother with whom one cannot positively identify, nor turn to for comfort under strain, severely impedes identity development for girls, in particular, who need positive female role models with whom to identify. Leah, for example, in desperately trying to live up to her mother's desire, became the thin person her mother longed to be. Unable in this way to achieve the love and maternal nourishment she sought, Leah grew thinner and thinner, her anorexic symptoms becoming the sign of insufficient nurturance. Rather than recognizing the need for a different type of "food," the family became angry at Leah for being so "difficult," thereby further depriving her of the nurturance she needed and leaving her flailing ever further towards madness.

Meeting with Leah and her parents helped me to recognize the familial dynamic in which she was caught. Much as with Ava, Leah depended on her father for nurturance, a provision that was only forthcoming to the extent that the mother's needs did not conflict. When I spoke to Leah about what I had observed, recognition of the familial context was at first unfathomable and seemed dangerous. Over time, however, Leah's ability to recognize her parents' limits helped her to negotiate greater peace with them and thereby to achieve greater care and consideration, which also attenuated her psychotic symptoms.

For children, survival depends on being able to access caretaking. In the absence of adequate caretaking, children can defer their own needs to those of their parents as a means for ensuring survival (Guntrip, 1989). Because women's survival needs have left them highly adapted to reading and responding to social cues, they can become overly enmeshed in meeting others needs and out of touch with their own feelings (Charles, 2011). That type of lack was precisely what left Ava and Leah ungrounded in their own experience, unable to build a coherent story through which to make sense of self or experience. Because of the essential link between parental care and identity development, disorganized attachment is associated with lack of coherence in autobiographical memory, resulting in conflicting narratives that are difficult to integrate into a cogent whole (Main & Hesse, 1990). The person who cannot integrate the disparate threads of meaning into a coherent life story is then unstable at the core and vulnerable to misreadings that assault or distort her sense of self. Unintegrated, fragments of experience tend to erupt in odd, incomprehensible ways, as gaps, intrusions, or symptoms that elude conscious understanding and so can be read as a mark of psychosis rather than trauma. Such misreadings can be destabilizing, thereby pushing the person toward psychosis rather than providing assistance in recognizing strengths and weaknesses, and learning to better navigate the social surround. Adaptive development is thereby further constrained and impeded.

When families resist recognizing the extent of the trauma that has taken place, it is difficult for the child to recognize the contexts within which an experience or symptom might be understandable. Family structures that are too enmeshed do not allow the child to discover her own truths. There is no external law, no third perspective from which to evaluate truth claims in relation to one's own experience or values (Muller, 2011). It is that perspective that psychoanalytic psychotherapy can afford, particularly important in a social context in which vulnerable individuals can be mis-read by the very institutions to which they turn for care. Perhaps most insidious in this regard is the idea that "insight" can be equated with "acceptance of one's illness." Too many individuals have suffered at the hands of professionals who wield diagnoses with heavy hands, seemingly unaware of how destructive even the best of intentions at times can be.

For example, during my early years of training, I worked with a young woman who was profoundly lost in relation to herself but seemed to have great creative potential. She described her role in the family as being used by her parents and brothers as an emotional outlet and sexual object, a pattern she played out in later relationships as well. My supervisor saw her as "borderline" in a way that evoked such disparagement from him that I found it difficult to keep her in mind as a whole human being. Fortunately for her, it was soon clear to me that I could not present this case to this supervisor without losing sight of the woman seeking my assistance. This dilemma haunted her. Like many women, each time Kate sought refuge in a psychiatric institution, she was rediagnosed with what seemed to be the "flavor of the month"; borderline, bipolar, histrionic; the diagnoses seemed to chronicle evolving conceptions of the disparagement of bright, creative, struggling young women rather than afford any useful assistance to her. To the contrary, when she was diagnosed with the then popular Multiple Personality Disorder, put into a group of MPD patients, and began to conform to the expectation and to organize her understanding of herself along the lines offered, *I* drew a line. Looking to the hospital for care and comfort was clearly killing her. I told her that in order to continue working with her, I needed her to recognize that the hospital did not solve but rather exacerbated her problems. If she could recognize that this "home" afforded greater destruction than comfort, than we might be able to envision a more supportive resource during times of strain. I think that she needed someone to stand up for her and say "This is not all you are. You are more than this. Please stop torturing yourself in this way and let's try to find respite during difficult times that does not leave you further depleted and estranged from yourself."

At the clinic where I worked at the time, Kate had originally introduced herself to me as "a creative person." That characterization was met with more disdain than respect by staff and, yet, it was true, although her early life had left her making use of her creativity in ways that undermined her development rather than furthering it. It took many years of hard work for Kate to begin to re-discover her potency and potential (see Charles, 2001, for further details). As it turned out, she *was* a creative person, something she was able to bring into fruition in ways that have brought her enjoyment, satisfaction, and recognition in her own chosen field. As I think back on those difficult years of our work together, I am most aware of the determination in me that helped me to tolerate what needed to be tolerated—including at times not knowing whether she would live or die—in order for Kate to begin to get her bearings and find her own way. That is what I try to impart to young people who I supervise, that our crazy faith in another's potential is often the only bedrock on which a life can be built.

For those whose stories have pushed them outside of the narrow margins of what is acceptable within the confines of the family story, truth and reality can be precious and precarious. Virginia, for example, had become increasingly dysregulated in relation to the story that could not be told. She described her mother as wonderful and loving, creating wonderful opportunities for enjoyment for her children. What she had not been able to tolerate, it seemed, was to face whatever might disturb that lovely family narrative. Virginia, much like Rhys's Antoinette, came from a privileged family with a history of preserving surface appearances, at times at the expense of the child's development. An extremely bright and talented young woman, Virginia's development had become increasingly waylaid in ways that the parents could not make sense of. By the time I met her, the parents' story had become one in which Virginia's "madness" was a tragic presumption. Their efforts to assist her, then, collided with her efforts to register her own story.

Initial engagements with the family took the form of painful confrontations between two stories utterly at odds with one another. When the mother appealed to the therapist to stop her daughter from attacking her, the response was an interpretive one, that Virginia seemed to be repeating a story that had not been able to register in either parent's mind. In this way, the therapist's assertion of the legitimacy of Virginia's perspective (that might be quite different from the mother's own) made it possible for two different stories to be told such that a conversation between two different minds might evolve. There are truths that are as difficult to hear as they might be to tell. For Virginia's parents, it was difficult to face the possibility that their child might have been injured while under their care. Their lack of recognition of the source of her distress left Virginia unable to recognize her own distress until a previous therapist had recognized symptoms of early trauma. That recognition afforded the grounding Virginia needed in order to begin to register and make sense of her symptoms.

Virginia's nascent recognition of the sources of her distress helped her to make better choices in spite of her disequilibrium. She was able to resist, for example, the diagnosis of schizophrenia when that was offered as a way of making sense of her symptoms that did not recognize the story behind the symptoms. At that juncture, Virginia was able to oppose the medicalized truth with the truth of her experience, insisting that the diagnosis did not make sense because it did not take into account her trauma history. That insistence helped Virginia find a therapist who recognized that the abuse history did make a difference in terms of how her story was told and how one might proceed. Putting together the story of her abuse and the ways in which her repression of that abuse had undermined her efforts to build a life became the foundation on which her identity could more solidly be built.

CONCLUSION

We live in an era in which different and opposing "truths" vie for our attention. In such an era, we can recognize the contextual nature of meanings, and ways in which meanings are built in relation to both individual and consensual experience. That recognition helps us to respectfully encounter those with very different world views and ways of describing their experience. Novelists offer us opportunities for such encounters. Elizabeth Bowen, for example, explores difficulties women face when social conventions preclude deeper, more open relational engagements. In her novels, she high-lights ways in which individuals can bump into one another without recognition, social niceties taking the place of actual engagement. Through her fine-ly drawn characters, one can recognize ways in which a woman can lose herself in relation to this impermeability of surface veneer that fails to ac-knowledge anything that threatens to disturb the polish. It is a polish that seems to serve as a mirror; characters rarely seem to be able to do other than encounter reflections of themselves. In such a universe, myopic Emmeline, who takes off her glasses in order to present a more pleasing face to others, is utterly unable to recognize ways in which she is being used by those she most trusts (Bowen, 1950). The fault lines in these relationships leave her bereft and then utterly mad, described by the author as an absence of the self that might recognize the injury and thereby suffer it, to endure and learn to bear painful truths. When survival becomes a forced choice between mad-ness and recognition of the inhumanity with which one is treated by those in whom one has placed one's trust, it may be better to go mad, to leave one's sensibilities behind and float in an interim space in which one is, for the moment, free from the pain of recognition of whatever truths are too terrible to bear.

I am, fundamentally, a humanist psychoanalyst. I hope to provide those I work with enough space and time to begin to confront themselves with increasing depth and complexity on their road toward becoming themselves. Increasingly, I see the work that we do in psychoanalysis and psychoanalytic psychotherapy as building reflective function, which, in turn, builds resil-ience. I have come to think of resilience as a marker for the types of meta-cognitive abilities so crucial to finding one's way in the world (see, for example, Fonagy, Gergely, Jurist, & Target, 2002; Lysaker et al., 2011). The ability to reflect on one's thoughts and feelings in relation to the thoughts and feelings of others involves capacities that are built over time through interac-tions in the social environment. For those who have receded from such interactions, trying to move beyond the point of impasse can feel impossible. My interest in psychosis and in creativity has led me to investigate ways in which psychosis may mark thwarted capacities that find their creative ex-pression in the symptom. From a psychoanalytic perspective, the symptom can be read as a communication from the unconscious that cannot be spoken more directly. Learning to read one's self and to be able to track one's thoughts is the work of psychoanalysis, as the person moves toward a more genuinely creative expression, a freer free association.

Recognizing that the symptom is also a metaphor also helps me to hold in mind a person's reality that may be very different from my own and yet might be workable for that individual. Part of what makes this type of hold-ing so important to me—so precious and so precarious—is the instability that can come with idiosyncracy, an instability that is not unfamiliar to me. I have long been interested in the at-times fine line between creativity and madness, trying to understand what might stabilize the idiosyncratic individual enough to be able to continue to be creative. My initial passion comes from my own struggles but has been fed by my empathic concern for those who have been less fortunate than myself and for whom life remains torturous.

Early in my training, I came upon the idea that there was a higher incidence of "colorful personalities" in families with higher incidences of psychosis, a link affirmed by more recent work, as well (Jackson, 2015). That link intrigued me and led to studies of creative individuals such as Van Gogh (Charles & Telis, 2014) and Virginia Woolf (Charles, 2015), who struggled to be highly idiosyncratic without losing their bearings. My research has helped me to better take a stand in my clinical work when confronted with individuals who have experienced psychotic symptoms but whose problems seem to stem largely from having had insufficient interactive containment to establish a coherent and stable identity.

In my experience, growth depends on our ability to be interested in the challenges we encounter so that we can look beyond the surface to deconstruct, recontextualize, and reconsider meanings. Whereas experiences of mastery enhance those capacities, fear, and shame each inhibit curiosity, collapsing the reflective space and closing down the potential for new learning. Learning requires our willingness to take apart the picture as we have known it and tolerate fragmentation so that integration might occur at a higher level.

One can only be free and creative to the extent that one can trust that there is an environment sufficiently safe and reliable on which to land. For those for whom interpersonal engagement has meant misrecognition, intrusion, neglect, and denial, engagement with another human being can be a dangerous proposition. I find that taking a stand regarding the possibility of meaning-making, as I try to offer the missing pieces as they emerge in the work, helps those I work with build a coherent narrative in which the fragments that could not be assimilated can come together into a more coherent form. Because emotional intensity can interfere with cognitive functions, attending to the level of distress helps to invite *repair* rather than retraumatization. Much as the attuned parent meets the child's affect and *only then* moves toward softening and soothing, we must be able to meet our patients where they are, even in moments of darkest despair or psychotic levels of disregulation. What we call psychosis is often a function of the panic—and shame—that ensues when we are pushed beyond our limits, our reflective capacities fail, and there is no one there (externally or internally) on whom to rely while we reconstitute. Abjection has an impact. As the clinician looks for patterns with interest, curiosity, and compassionate respect, we model a more facilitative mode of tolerating failure as we struggle with complex difficulties.

Trauma disrupts mind and memory, and meanings can become concrete and unwieldy. Metaphors afford a means for communicating experience that is largely ineffable and beyond words, and also for holding hope. Metaphors breathe life into the work because they are, of essence, play*ful*: they cannot be taken in directly, but rather must be *played with*. There is an essential dialectic between processes of fragmentation and integration that Winnicott (1971) points to in the *use of an object*. In order to be able to interact with another person as a separate and sentient being, we must learn that the other can survive our attempts to differentiate ourselves, even if these *feel* destructive. We need to be able to bump into one another, leave an imprint, and back away and try to get some perspective on the encounter.

Psychoanalytic psychotherapy can perhaps best be likened to a dance. As we interplay, over time, with one another, we are building meanings together. For those for whom trauma or neglect has fundamentally impeded their self-development, leaving them at risk of psychotic experience, we need to be able to register meanings through our feelings as well as through our words. Respectfully engaging at the sensory level helps us to build metaphors that do not violate the experience. Much as the clinician needs to be able to tune her sensibilities, her *instrument*, if you will; so, too, Ava needed to become familiar with her own. She began to wander down to the shop, where she played at drawing. Ava—whose perfectionism and attention to external markers of value make it difficult for her to discover her own— imagined being able to surmount the impasse by doing "bad art," likely a brilliant move on her part. As she struggles with writing, getting lost behind ideas of good writing that leave her unable to write, I suggest she engage with her writing like a squiggle game, hoping she might be able to become interested in her own productions. As she tries my ideas on for size, she is able, at times, to find her way into the playfulness through which she might develop her potential. Now, when she returns home, Ava at times feels as though she is losing her mind. At this point, however, we have the benefit of all that we have learned about Ava and her past, and can use this experience as a way of empathizing with the plight Ava had been in as a young child in similar confrontations. Recognizing the dynamic rather than entirely becoming lost in it once again helps Ava to re-find herself, separate and apart from her mother, rather than becoming lost, once again, within her mother's distress and confusion.

Identity develops within the narratives between parent and child. The child pieces together the threads of being through the bits and fragments of experience as they are internalized. With sufficient stability, the bits are woven together into an identity that can withstand the assaults of daily experience. The lesson we must all learn from the attachment literature is to recognize that incoherence in self-narrative and identity has to do with development gone awry. And development gone awry needs attention to development, beginning at the point of the rupture. At Riggs, when we are having a particularly difficult time with a patient and discussing our struggles in team meetings, I tend to wonder aloud how young the particular behavioral dynamic might be. Being able to recognize the two-, three-, or twelve-year-old within the adult, who is seeking resolution to a very real developmental impasse, can help us to more empathically recognize the fault lines and attend to them. We are all, indeed, *"much more simply human than otherwise"* (Sullivan, 1953, p. 32; italics in original), and it can be difficult to recognize extreme trauma and feel empathically tied to it. And yet, it is in our deepest connections to one another that healing happens.

Stories can provide a means for justifying what should not be justified but can also provide a means for exploring the complexities of existence through another lens. We are, inherently, storied individuals, developing our identities through the narratives exchanged between parent and child and then with one another as the years go by. Social values and prejudice find their way into our stories, and it behooves us to reflect actively on ways in which the stories, as we have come to know them, contribute to or foreclose the development of our fellow beings. The woman's story has been insufficiently written. I hope that this deficit will be remedied as women continue to write their own stories in counterpoint to those of the men, as we all struggle to make room for the full range of possibilities within ourselves and, in this way, enhance our creative potential and our ability to live well in our own lives and with one another.

REFERENCES

Abraham, N. (1975). Notes on the Phantom: A Complement to Freud's Metapsychology. In: N. Abraham & M. Torok, M. (1994). *The Shell and the Kernel*, pp. 171–76. N. T. Rand (Ed. & Trans.). Chicago & London: University of Chicago Press.

Abraham, N., & Torok, M. (1994). *The Shell and the Kernel.* N. T. Rand (Ed. & Trans.). Chicago & London: University of Chicago Press.

Apprey, M. (1993). The African-American Experience: Forced Migration and the Transgenerational Trauma. *Mind and Human Interaction*, 4:70–75.

Atkinson, J. (2002). *Trauma Trails, Recreating Song Lines: The Transgenerational Effects of Trauma in Indigenous Australia.* North Melbourne: Spinifex Press.

Ayral-Clause, O. (2002). *Camille Claudel: A Life.* New York: Abrams.

Bakhtin, M. (1981). *The Dialogic Imagination.* (M. Holquist, Ed.; C. Emerson & M. Holquist, Trans.). Austin: University of Texas Press.

Belenky, M. F., Clinchy, B. M., Goldberger, N. R., & Tarule, J. M. (1986). *Women's Ways of Knowing: The Development of Self, Voice, and Mind.* New York: Basic Books.

Bion, W.R. (1977). *Seven Servants*, New York: Jason Aronson.

Bowen, E. (1950). *To the North.* New York: Alfred Knopf.

Breuer, J., & Freud, S. (1893-1895). *Studies on Hysteria.* In: S. Freud, *The Standard Edition of the Complete Psychological Works of Sigmund Freud.* London: Hogarth Press, 1971.

Brontë, C. (2006). *Jane Eyre.* London: Penguin Classics.

Bucci, W. (2001). Pathways of Emotional Communication. *Psychoanalytic Inquiry,* 21:40–70.

Busfield, J. (1988). Mental Illness as Social Product or Social Construct: A Contradiction in Feminists' Arguments? *Sociology of Health and Illness,* 10:521–42.

Carlisle, L. V. (2010). *Elizabeth Packard: A Noble Fght*. Urbana and Chicago: University of Illinois Press.

Charles, M. (2000). Convex and Concave, Part I: Images of Emptiness in Women. *American Journal of Psychoanalysis*, 60(1): 5–28.

Charles, M. (2001). Reflections on Creativity: The "Intruder" as Mystic OR Reconciliation with the Mother/Self. *Free Associations*, 9(1:49):119–51.

Charles, M (2004). Women and Psychotherapy on Film: Shades of Scarlett Conquering. In J. R. Brandell (Ed.), *Celluloid Couches, Cinematic Clients: Psychoanalysis and Psychotherapy in the Movies*. Albany: SUNY Press.

Charles, M. (2011). What Does a Woman Want? *Psychoanalysis, Culture, and Society*, 16(4):337–53.

Charles, M. (2013). Bullying and Social Exclusion: Links to Severe Psychopathology. In M. O'Loughlin (Ed.), *Working with Children's Emotional Lives: Psychodynamic Perspectives on Children and Schools*, New York: Jason Aronson, pp. 207–26.

Charles, M. (2014a). The Intergenerational Transmission of Trauma: Effects on Identity Development. In N. Tracey (Ed.). *Transgenerational Trauma and the Aboriginal Preschool Child: Healing through Intervention*. Lanham, MD: Rowman & Littlefield, pp. 133–52.

Charles, M. (2014b). Trauma, Childhood, and Emotional Resilience. In N. Tracey (Ed.). *Transgenerational Trauma and the Aboriginal Preschool Child: Healing through Intervention*. Lanham, MD: Rowman & Littlefield, pp. 109–31.

Charles, M. (2015). *Psychoanalysis and Literature: The Stories We Live*. New York: Rowman & Littlefield.

Charles, M., Clemence, J., & Biel, S. (2011). Psychosis and Creativity: Managing Cognitive Complexity on Unstructured Tasks. In: L. DellaPietra (ed.), *Perspectives on Creativity, Volume II*, pp. 107–22. Newcastle upon Tyne: Cambridge Scholars Publishing.

Charles, M., Durham-Fowler, J., & Malone, J. (2016). Factors that Discriminate Creative Engagement on an Unstructured Task: Creativity and the Rorschach. *Bulletin of the Menninger Clinic*, 80: 97–130.

Charles, M., Frank, S. J., Jacobson, S., & Grossman, G. (2001). Repetition of the Remembered Past: Patterns of Separation-Individuation in Two Generations of Mothers and Daughters. *Psychoanalytic Psychology*, 18:705–28.

Charles, M., & O'Loughlin, M. (2013). The Complex Subject of Psychosis. Special Issue: Psychosis, M. Charles, Guest Editor. *Psychoanalysis, Culture, and Society*, 17(4):410–21.

Charles, M. & Telis, K. (2014). Pattern as Inspiration and Mode of Communication in the Works of Van Gogh. In: M. G. Fromm (Ed.), *A Spirit that Impels: Play, Creativity, and Psychoanalysis*. London: Karnac, pp. 95–121.

Chesler, P. (1972). *Women and Madness*. New York: Doubleday.

Collins, R. (Director/Producer). (2000). *We Don't Live Under Normal Conditions* [Video]. United States: Fanlight Productions.

Davoine, F., & Gaudillière, J. M. (2004). *History Beyond Trauma* (trans. S. Fairfield). New York: Other.

de Lauretis, T. (1984). *Alice Doesn't: Feminism, Semiotics, Cinema*. Bloomington: Indiana University Press.

Diamond, M. J. (2004). The Shaping of Masculinity: Revisioning Boys Turning Away from their Mothers to Construct a Male Gender Identity. *International Journal of Psychoanalysis*, 85:359–80.

Dimen, M. (2003). *Sexuality, Intimacy, Power*. Hillsdale, NJ: Analytic Press.

Edwards, R. (2011). Women's and Gender History. In E. Foner & L. McGirr (Eds), *American History Now*. Philadelphia: Temple University Press, pp. 336–53.

Eliot, G. (1963) *Essays of George Eliot*. T. Pinney (Ed.). London: Routledge & Kegan Paul.

Fivush, R., Habermas, T., Waters, T. E. A., & Zaman, W. (2011). The making of autobiographical memory: Intersections of culture, narratives and identity. *New International Journal of Psychology*, 46:321–45.

Fonagy, P., Gergely, G., Jurist, E. L., & Target, M. (2002). *Affect Regulation, Mentalization, and the Development of the Self*. New York: Other.

Forrest, W. C. (1969). Literature as Aesthetic Object: The Kinesthetic Stratum. *The Journal of Aesthetics and Art Criticism.* 27(4):455–59.

Gallese, V. (2009). Mirror Neurons, Embodied Simulation, and the Neural Basis of Social Identification. *Psychoanalytic Dialogues,* 19:519–36.

Geller, J. L., & Harris, M. (1994) *Women of the Asylum: Voices from Behind the Walls, 1840-1945.* New York: Doubleday.

Ghent, E. (1990). Masochism, Submission, Surrender: Masochism as a Perversion for Surrender. *Contemporary Psychoanalysis,* 26:108–36.

Gilligan, C. & Richards, D. A. J. (2009). *The Deepening Darkness: Patriarchy, Resistance, and Democracy's Future.* Cambridge: Cambridge University Press.

Guntrip, H. (1989). *Schizoid Phenomena, Object-Relations and the Self.* Madison, CT: International Universities Press.

Hammersley, P., Read, J., Woodall, S., & Dillon, J. (2007). Childhood trauma and psychosis: The genie is out of the bottle. *Journal of Psychological Trauma,* 6:7-20.

Hirschbein, L. (2010). Sex and Gender in Psychiatry: A View from History. *Journal of Medical Humanities,* 31:155-170.

Hornstein, G. A. (2009). *Agnes's Jacket: A Psychologist's Search for the Meanings of Madness.* New York: Rodale.

Hutcheson, J. (1983). Subdued Feminism, Jane Austen, Charlotte Brontë and George Eliot. *International Journal of Women's Studies,* 6:230–57.

Jackson, M. (2015). *Creativity and Psychotic States in Exceptional People* (J. Magagna, Ed.). *London:* Routledge.

Jackson, P. L., Meltzoff, A. N., & Decety, J. (2006). Neural Circuits Involved in Imitation and Perspective-Taking. *NeuroImage,* 31:429–39.

Kavanaugh, P. B. (2012). *Stories from the Bog: On Madness, Philosophy, and Psychoanalysis.* Amsterdam & New York: Rodopi.

Klein, M. (1975). Notes on some Schizoid Mechanisms. In *Envy and Gratitude and Other Works, 1946–1963* (pp. 1–24). London: Hogarth Press.

Kilintari, M., Narayana, S., Babajani-Feremi, A., Rezai, R., & Papanicolaou, A. C. (2016). Brain Activation Profiles During Kinesthetic and Visual Imagery: An fMRI Study. *Brain Research,* 1646:249–61.

Krasner, L. (2016). *Women of Abstract Expressionism.* Denver Art Museum, Denver, CO.

LaCapra, D. (1999). Trauma, Absence, Loss. *Critical Inquiry,* 25:696–727.

Layton, L. (2004). Relational No More: Defensive Autonomy in Middle-Class Women. *Annual of Psychoanalysis,* 32:29–42.

Light, A. (Director), & Saraf, I. (Producer). (1993). *Dialogues with Madwomen* [Video]. United States: Light-Saraf Films.

Liotti, G. (2004). Trauma, Dissociation, and Disorganized Attachment: Three Strands of a Single Braid. *Psychotherapy: Theory, Research, Practice, Training,* 41:472–86.

Longden, E., & Read, J. (2016). Social Adversity in the Etiology of Psychosis: A Review of the Evidence. *American Journal of Psychotherapy,* 70:5–33.

Lynam, M. J., & Cowley, S. (2007). Understanding Marginalization as a Social Determinant of Health. *Critical Public Health,* 17:137–49.

Lysaker, P.H., Olesek, K. L., Warman, D. M., Martin, J. M., Salzman, A. K., Nicolò. G., Salvatore, G., & Dimaggio, G. (2011). Metacognition in Schizophrenia: Correlates and Stability of Deficits in Theory of Mind and Self-reflectivity. *Psychiatry Research,* 190:18–22.

Machann, C. (2005). The Male Villain as Domestic Tyrant in *Daniel Deronda:* Victorian Masculinities and the Cultural Context of George Eliot's Novel. *Journal of Men's Studies,* 13:327–46.

Main, M. & Hesse, E. (1990). Parent's Unresolved Traumatic Experiences are Related to Infant Disorganized/disoriented Attachment Status: Is Frightened and/or Frightening Parental Behavior the Linking Mechanism? In: M. Greenberg, D. Cicchetti, & E. M. Cummings (Eds.), *Attachment in the Preschool Years: Theory, Research, and Intervention* (pp. 161–82). Chicago: University of Chicago Press.

Mar, R. A., & Oatley, K. (2008). The Function of Fiction is the Abstraction and Simulation of Social Experience. *Perspectives on Psychological Science*, 3:173–92.

Marter, J. (2016). *Women of Abstract Expressionism*. New Haven, CT:Yale University Press.

Miall, D. S., & Kuiken, D. (1994). Beyond Text Theory: Understanding Literary Response. *Discourse Processes*, 17:337–52.

Miller, J. B. (1976). *Towards a New Psychology of Women*. Boston: Random House.

Morton, T. A., Haslam, S. A., Postmes, T., & Hornsey, M. J. (2009). Theorizing Gender in the Face of Social Change: Is There Anything Essential about Essentialism? *Journal of Personality and Social Psychology*, 96:653–64.

Muller, J. (2011). Why the Pair needs the Third. In: E. M. Plakun (Ed.), *Treatment Resistance and Patient Authority: The Austen Riggs Reader*, pp. 97–120. New York: W. W. Norton.

Murphy, T. A. (2013). *Citizenship and the Origins of Women's History in the United States*. Philadelphia: University of Pennsylvania Press.

Netjek, V. A., Allison, N., & Hilburn, C. (2012). Race- and Gender-related Difference in Clinical Characteristics and Quality of Life among Outpatients with Psychotic Disorders. *Journal of Psychiatric Practice*, 18:329–37.

Paris, R.-M. (1988). *Camille: The Life of Camille Claudel, Rodin's Muse and Mistress*. New York: Holt.

Parkes, C. M., Stevensen-Hinde, J., & Maris, P. (1991). *Attachment Across the Life Cycle*. London: Routledge.

Pheterson, G. (2009). Alliances between Women: Overcoming Internalized Oppression and Internalized Domination In. L. Albrecht & R. Brewer (Eds.), *Bridges of Power: Women's Multicultural Alliances* (pp. 34–48). Philadelphia: New Society Publishers.

Rhys, J. (1966). *Wide Sargasso Sea*. New York: W. W. Norton.

Seikkula, J., & Olson, M. E. (2003). The Open Dialogue Approach to Acute Psychosis: Its Poetics and Micropolitics. *Family Process*, 42:403–18.

Sullivan, H. S. (1953). *The Interpersonal Theory of Psychiatry*. New York: William Alanson White Psychiatric Foundation.

Tappan, M. B. (2005). Domination, Subordination and the Dialogic Self: Identity Development and the Politics of "Ideological Becoming." *Culture & Psychology*, 11:47–75.

Tappan, M. B. (2006). Reframing Internalized Oppression and Internalized Domination: From the Psychological to the Sociocultural. *Teachers College Record*, 108:2115–144.

Thomas, S. P. (2005). Women's Anger, Aggression, and Violence. *Health Care for Women International*, 26:504–22.

Tomkins. S. S. (1982). Affect Theory. In P. Ekman, W. V. Friesen. & P. Ellsworth (Eds.). *Emotion in the Human Face* (2nd ed.), pp. 353–405. Cambridge: Cambridge University Press.

Van Buren, J. (1994). The Engendering of Female Subjectivity. *American Journal of Psychoanalysis*, 54:109–25.

van Ijzendoorn, M. H., Schuengel, C., & Bakermans-Kranenburg, M. J. (1999). Disorganized Attachment in Early Childhood: Meta-analysis of Precursors, Concomitants, and Sequelae. *Development and Psychopathology*, 11:225–49.

Walker, J. (1994). Psychoanalysis and Feminist Film Theory: The Problem of Sexual Difference and Identity. In D. Carson, L. Dittmar, & J. R. Welsh (Eds.), *Multiple Voices in Feminist film Criticism* (pp. 82–92). Minneapolis: University of Minnesota Press.

Winnicott, D. W. (1971). *Playing and Reality*. London: Hogarth Press.

Woodman, D., & Wyn, J. (2015). Class, Gender and Generation Matter: Using the Concept of Social Generation to Study Inequality and Social Change. *Journal of Youth Studies*, 18:1402–410.

Woolf, V. (1928). *Orlando: A Biography*. London: Hogarth Press.

Woolf, V. (1929). *A Room of One's Own*. London: Hogarth Press.

NOTE

1. All of the names used in this book are pseudonyms.

Chapter Two

Explicate or Relate

Recognizing and Differentiating Literary Madwomen

Helen DeVinney

It was my ninth-grade English teacher who asked: are we sure Alice is dreaming in Lewis Carroll's *Alice in Wonderland*, or might it be a delusion? While her madness seemed harmless in dream-form, I remember feeling uncomfortable thinking about what it would mean if these were ideas in her waking, perhaps, psychotic thoughts. This same English teacher shocked us all again while reading *Jane Eyre*, when she suggested that perhaps the described madwoman, Bertha, might not seem so crazy if we considered Bertha's point of view. The challenge of that thought stirred shame in me: I had not hesitated to accept the portrait of Bertha. It had never occurred to me to question that not only was it possible that Jane's perception was flawed and second-hand, but that it did not consider Bertha's subjective experience.

After high school, I continued to be fascinated by the number of stories that included "crazy" characters, and it became quickly obvious that the vast majority of those characters were female. As an undergraduate student majoring in English and Classical Studies, I seemed surrounded by female characters whose sense of reality could not be trusted, whose delusions of grandeur and desire for omnipotent power led them to violence, and whose greatness could only be seen when chastened with accompanying insanity. At times, the prevalence of insanity in female characters felt so ubiquitous, I ceased to even register it as notable. Later, in a doctoral English program, I studied theories of race, gender, sexuality, and class alongside literature, and I began to observe the way in which a female character's relationship to privilege directly corresponded to the ways her "crazy" might be seen by other characters, by readers, and by literary critics. Since beginning work as a psychologist, I haven't found the gendered representation of "crazy" to be much different; there are countless "stories" told by therapists, and the vast majority of the "crazy" characters are women. When I worked in an inpatient hospital, women with psychosis were shrugged off as "crazy" in a way that many men with psychosis were not—they were quicker to be seen as malingering or psychopathic.

The more experience I gained as a clinician, the more my thoughts returned to these "crazy" female characters. From Classical times to the present, in different cultures and contexts, our stories return again and again to women who appear "crazy"—Cassandra in Aeschylus's *Agamemnon,* Ophelia in Shakespeare's *Hamlet*, Cathy Earnshaw in Emily Brontë's *Wuthering Heights*, Bertha Mason in Charlotte Brontë's *Jane Eyre*, Emma Bovary in Gustav Flaubert's *Madame Bovary*, The Protagonist of "The Yellow Wallpaper," and Sethe in Toni Morrison's *Beloved*, to name only a few. Why? What do we make of these "crazy" women, the re-occurring madwoman? To understand female characters who appear "crazy" requires a willingness to step into the mess. Rebecca Solnit writes in her 2017 essay, "A Short History of Silence" that part of how we make the world in which we live is through the shared task of "calling things by their true names" (p. 73). To this end, let us investigate the world we make with the words we use to describe these characters and determine whether or not madness is the "true name" of these characters.

Words like "crazy," "mad," "insane," "psychotic," and "delusional" are often used interchangeably. What do we learn by the origin of these words, their associations, and their use in the vernacular? Are there ways we might better understand the purpose or function of such characters simply by delving further into the language that is used to describe both the characters themselves and their experiences?

Second, we must consider how feminist criticism has responded to the literary madwoman and how that response has evolved over time, particularly as feminist theory has struggled to both free itself of internalized misogyny and to incorporate intersectional thinking. Approaching these female characters (and sexism more generally) intersectionally is key, as confusion and disagreement have resulted from efforts to offer universalist readings of women's oppression in literature. While well-intentioned, eliding important differences around race, class, and sexuality effectively bring the conversation to a halt. The sometimes failure to recognize differences in the experiences of female characters who appear "crazy" is yet another form of silencing that must be exposed.

MEANINGS AND ASSOCIATIONS, EXPLICIT AND IMPLICIT

Terms like "crazy," "mad," and "insane," are all shorthand for suggesting that someone is psychotic or is in acting in a way that is consistent with a psychotic process. Understanding the etymological root of these words often helps us to uncover some of the meanings and associations concealed in the words. The term "psychosis" originates from the Greek "psykhe" and "osis," meaning "mind" and "abnormal condition." Interestingly, the Greek word "psykhosis" meant a "giving of life" or "animation." Thus, in the word's etymological roots, we see this duality, a meaning at once of abnormal thinking and invigoration. These multiple meanings capture the sometimes very complex inner world of persons experiencing psychosis who may at once may feel frustration at not being able to organize their thinking while simultaneously feeling an incredible rush of creativity or generativity.

Before moving away from etymology and meaning, we might consider the word "mad." The word appears to date back to the late thirteenth century from Old English, and its earliest forms, *gemæded* and *gemædan* mean "rendered insane" and "to make insane or foolish." What is interesting about the etymology of the word is that woven into its meaning is the sense that the "insane" state is the result of some kind of outside pressure—one has been "rendered" or "made" to be in this state. Certainly, this connotation is preserved in the colloquial sense of feeling "driven mad." In considering female characters who are mad, as will be discussed in detail, many of the characters find themselves in situations in which we may wonder about to what extent they would be able to maintain sanity; or, are the conditions of their environment such that remaining "sane" (from the Latin, "healthy") would actually be the sign of insanity? Is their distress, in fact, normative in their conditions?

The woman who is driven "mad" is devalued not only because of her identity (gender, race, etc.) but also because of her mental illness; yet, her illness also brings a strange kind of power; she is "marked" as a woman who is unpredictable, who defies societal standards and pressures. In this way, she creates fear in others. In noticing the prevalence of women "going crazy," we might wonder about the power available to women. Women struggle to find ways to make their voices heard, and many women in the present day discover that engaging in the same strategies that would be not only accepted but respected in men earn them further marginalization and scorn. Women often find themselves struggling with a message that they are to be less emotional and sensitive if they want to be taken seriously and then told they need to less shrill and demanding if they want to be heard. It is no wonder that in slipping into madness, women may feel some freedom, as they lose the yoke of having to calculate how to present themselves and just bring their mess unapologetically. But the freedom is a qualified one, because for whatever voice madness yields, the marginalization of mental illness still renders the crazy woman silent.

READING THE MADWOMAN TO ACCOUNT FOR MULTIPLE MINORITY IDENTITIES

In understanding why women are often experienced or dismissed as crazy, we might take a moment just to think through the inevitable consequences of a patriarchal societal. In a society that has a clear power hierarchy, the group with the most power and privilege tends to reject or minimize those characteristics or qualities that threaten their ability to maintain power. Traits such as weakness, emotionality, sensitivity, and vulnerability are seen as liabilities, and so they are disavowed in the group with power (i.e., white men in Western contexts), and are instead seen as defining characteristics in the group without power (i.e., women). This creates a paradox where these defining characteristics are both used as a justification for why women cannot be the ruling demographic and exist as coveted traits that men want but can't have without risking their status; thus, by a trick of their own hands, men feel burdened by the need to maintain power and envious of fuller ranges of expression that threaten that power. Men learn not to identify or express qualities considered feminine; to confirm their masculinity, they disavow these "weak" traits and embrace hyper-masculinity. Because men must sacrifice qualities deemed feminine to retain power, men may feel envious of these expressed traits in women. This can stir in men vengeful and violent feelings toward women, unconsciously feeling that if they cannot have tenderness and vulnerability for themselves, then no one will.

Perhaps there is no more obvious example of the hegemonic underpinnings of the connection between madness and women than the fact that the specter of the madwoman invites a propensity toward monolithic thinking, even amongst feminists. It can be easy to slip into a pattern in which one imagines a sameness in women's experiences that allows for one woman's madness and its meaning to be interchangeable with another woman's madness, despite differences in race, class, sexuality and context. In this way, a crazy woman is never unique but rather a variation on a theme. Exploring an individual madwoman's story is often eclipsed by a universal story that draws sweeping conclusions about women and society. We argue over whether or not madness can be used to subvert patriarchy and constructions of gender, sometimes failing to note that the answer to that question depends on the woman herself, because even within the category of woman there are differences in privilege.

If one wants to discuss madness in female literary characters, it is impossible not to reference Sandra Gilbert and Susan Gubar's text, *The Madwoman in the Attic* (1979). For most readers and critics alike, this was the first text to provide a large-scale conversation about the representation of female characters as mad. And while the text brought much-needed attention to these overlooked literary figures, it also presented an argument that was in-line with what is now called "white feminism," which is that when talking about the oppression of women, it does so in a way that fails to note how differences in race, class, and sexuality might make those experiences of oppression vastly different. Gilbert and Gubar saw the category of gender as something that was unifying for women. Their thesis implicitly presupposed that regardless of race, sexuality, or class, gender was the most important aspect of identity, implying a sameness that makes one woman's struggle representative of all women's struggles.

To illustrate the problem of Gilbert and Gubar's approach, we might look at their treatment of the titular madwoman, Bertha Mason of *Jane Eyre*. The authors discuss Bertha as a split-off aspect of both the character, Jane, and Brontë herself. In these discussions, issues of race and class are completely elided. Bertha Mason, is a Creole woman transplanted to England to marry Rochester, a white man with privileges related to his gender, race, and class. In fact, the marriage itself can be seen as an enactment and reflection of colonialism in the Caribbean. Bertha is in a very different situation than Jane and to ignore the disparities between them is a function of white privilege. In referring to Bertha as the shadow of both Jane and Brontë herself, Gilbert and Gubar suggest that Bertha's experience of oppression as a Creole woman brought to England by marriage is synonymous with that of white women indigenous to England who have the benefits of race, culture, and class/education. Of course, the problem with this false equivalency is that Bertha's ethnic identity alone renders her of even less social and political status than almost any white British woman. Moreover, Bertha is not just socially, creatively and psychically confined but is literally locked in an attic. Brontë herself participates in perpetuating racial stereotypes of her day, as her violent, wild, crazy representation of herself is, not coincidentally, a woman of color; while likely unconscious, it is not meaningless that the mad woman is Creole. This is not to diminish the struggles of nineteenth-century white women, but to suggest that their experiences of oppression are interchangeable with Bertha's is simply false. In the rush for solidarity and in overlooking their own privilege, some Western, white feminists still fail to make space for the fact that women of color, women from developing nations, and women whose religion, sexuality, and politics place them in the margins, experience sexism differently than Western, white women with majority identifications.

In the case of Bertha specifically, this more intersectional view seeks to factor other aspects of identity into the context of her experience of madness. Additionally, the emergence of mental health advocacy and disability studies have also helped to reveal other aspects of the universalizing aspects of Gilbert and Gubar's argument. Activists in the more medical-model mental health advocacy community take issue with ways of reading madness as *only* a form of protest or resistance, which complicates and/or erases the possible organic markers and physiological aspects of mental illness. From a related but different perspective, those in disability studies also question why "madness" by necessity must dictate it as "other," encouraging readers to think about another invisible layer of oppression that presupposes those who present as different (mentally or physically) must be necessarily impaired. [1]

To provide some context for Gilbert and Gubar's use of madness, we might consider the work of Phyllis Chesler. Prior to the publication of *The Madwoman in the Attic*, psychologist Phyllis Chesler authored *Women and Madness* (1972), in which she explored a "double sexual standard of mental health," arguing that standards of mental health are gendered male, inviting a binary in which mental illness would thus be gendered female (p. 56). As Schlichter (2003) observes, the foundation of Chesler's argument was built on critiques of psychoanalysis and psychiatry by pioneers of feminism, such as Betty Friedan, who argued that these systems provided an infrastructure for oppressing women by categorizing them as insane or hysterical. In turn, Chesler's work paved the way for feminists to problematize representations of mad women as "ill," with many feminist critics beginning to see madness as a way for women to exploit the system pointed against them; madness was read as a way to rebel and resist patriarchy.

It is from this place of "madness-as-rebellion" that Gilbert and Gubar (1979) grounded their argument. They focused less on the female characters as agents of rebellion or subversion, and more on how the female authors used their characters as representations of the parts of themselves they had to suppress and disavow in order to make their way in society and, more specifically, in the male-dominated world of writing and publishing. The book's main thesis and the title itself borrows from Charlotte Brontë's *Jane Eyre*, in which the character of Bertha Mason is confined to the attic. Within the narrative of the novel, the reader is led to believe that there is no choice but to lock Bertha away because her madness renders her a danger to herself and others. Bertha's aggression toward Jane and her husband, Rochester, is seen as purely symptomatic of her "madness." While Gilbert and Gubar highlight the significance of Bertha's madness as resistance, they do not see her as the clearly racialized, postcolonial woman that she is and instead focus on her as a representation of the parts all women must keep "locked away." Gilbert and Gubar's argument implies that Bertha Mason has no agency of her own; she is the shadow side of Jane and Brontë herself.

This merger of Bertha-Jane-Brontë is notable for many reasons, not the least of which is a shift in focus, moving the discourse away from the representation of women in texts and extending it to the women writing the texts.

While attention to the struggle of female writers in the nineteenth century was important and groundbreaking work, Gilbert and Gubar's shift in focus, and their interpretation of Bertha as the messy, angry part of all women writers, is problematic. In seeing Bertha as "the shadow," they strip her of her own identity and instantly yoke together all women as a uniform, trans-historical category facing a shared experience of oppression and with a shared or identical shadow side. Gilbert and Gubar (1979) argue there is "a common, female impulse to struggle free from social and literary confine-ment through strategic redefinitions of self, art, and society" (p. xii). While Gilbert and Gubar deserve much credit for the attention they brought to how women are represented in literature, particularly in the nineteenth century, the idea that there is a universal female impulse is both an overgeneralization and an erasure of the very real disparities between women and their experi-ences that are the direct result of differences in race, class, sexuality and culture.

Many feminists of color have critiqued this collapsing of difference. In "Age, Race, Class, and Sex: Women Redefining Difference," Audre Lorde (1984) sought to help white feminists better understand the necessity of acknowledging differences. While this critique was first experienced as a way to separate woman from woman, a closer reading shows Lorde arguing against conflations because it is the insistence on sameness that causes feel-ings of separation. Lorde notes that when women refuse to acknowledge their differences, ruptures in understanding occur that lead to increased feelings of difference and isolation. By acknowledging variability in context, women can make space for the ways in which they do have a sense of a shared cause. While the category of woman is one that can be shared, and can be a source of solidarity, within that category are women who are white, of color, cis-gender, trans, gay, poor, wealthy, "crazy," and "sane," among other differ-ences. To suggest that women of such varied backgrounds and identities would experience oppression in the same way and would seek to subvert power in the same ways does not make sense. Neither oppression nor resis-tance is experienced uniformly across all women, is essential to any discus-sion of the madwoman in literature, as madness and its meaning work differ-ently depending on the degree of power, privilege, and voice the madwoman currently holds.

VARIABILITY IN PSYCHOSIS

A final consideration that we must explore before revisiting how we might better approach female characters who present as "mad" is to also highlight the way that madness itself is presented in a monolithic way. Women charac-ters are seen as going "crazy" or are described as "mad," as though the experience of psychosis is universal. Even within the medical model, psychotic processes are not contained in a single diagnosis. While schizophrenia is perhaps the best known psychotic illness, it is not the only one. Schizophrenia, as it is understood by Western medicine, is a chronic illness in which the person most often experiences visual or audio hallucinations and bizarre ideas without remission, and it is typically regarded as lasting from the time of onset to the end of the lifetime. Psychotic symptoms are also part of schizoaffective disorder, brief psychotic episodes, and substance-induced psychoses. Symptoms of psychosis can also be part of bipolar I disorder, major depression, and post-traumatic stress disorder. To suggest that these various forms and expressions of psychosis are interchangeable is inaccurate; in the same way we must understand different aspects of identity in order to understand each woman, so too must we understand the type of psychosis she is experiencing.

Also of note, in Western cultures, illnesses that are characterized by psychotic symptoms are largely thought to result from a combination of genetics, environment and individual temperament. This bio-psycho-social model has meant to serve as an answer to those who have been critical of the predominantly biological model, particularly as many biologically-based illnesses are chiefly treated through medications. Despite the acknowledgment of factors beyond biology, the bio-psycho-social model still places a heavy emphasis on genetics as it relates to causality. As such, some psychiatrists and researchers have begun to reemphasize the importance of social oppression and trauma in the development of psychotic symptomatology. The second edition of *Models of Madness* (2013), edited by John Read and Jacqui Dillons, discusses two important points: 1) there are different ways of understanding how psychosis develops and 2) the presence of hallucinations and delusions are chiefly the result of adverse life events, which is to say that abuse, oppression, and trauma are all conditions that often precede the onset of psychotic symptoms. With this in mind, it begs the question as to whether or not it continues to fit to diagnose someone with, say, schizophrenia, when there is evidence to suggest that the psychotic symptoms may directly related to an individual's experience of trauma. Because if trauma was a likely antecedent to psychosis and the psychosis is in response to trauma, does it not follow that the psychosis may *not* be unrelenting? Is it possible that by removing oneself from toxic situations and addressing trauma-related psychic-wounds that, in some cases, psychosis could largely resolve?

REVISITING THE MADWOMAN

As American Tibetan Buddhist nun Pema Chödrön writes in *When Things Fall Apart: Heart Advice for Difficult Times* (2000), "nothing ever goes away until it has taught us what we need to know" (p. 66). Rather than trying to explain the literary madwoman, might we consider *why* she appears—and why she continues to appear. In order to set the stage for an alternate discussion of what is being worked through in the repeated appearance of the madwoman, I would like to put three ideas in conversation: 1) R. D. Laing's hypothesis that what sometimes presents as psychotic behavior is in fact the collapse of what he calls the false self; 2) Northrop Frye's idea of a "recognition scene," and 3) the behavior Rebecca Solnit first described in her essay, "Men Explain Things to Me," now popularized as "mansplaining."

THE DIVIDED SELF

In *The Divided Self*, R. D. Laing (1960) argues that the collapse of reality inherent in psychosis results from entrapment in a false self. Laing's idea was that individuals often forsake internal authentic experiences in order to maintain order in the external system. The individual creates a false sense of self in order to maintain equilibrium in their environment. By societal standards or familial norms, this false self may appear "sane." However, if the individual cannot or will not maintain this false self and instead begins to act more authentically, those close to the individual would witness a sudden change in behavior that could be startling and even appear "crazy" to others.

For Laing, madness is always a response to environment. Laing suggests that the sudden onset of psychosis is really the true self casting off the shackles of the false self, which would feel like a sudden change to those in the system (p. 147). Laing argues that appearing "sane" within a sick system (via a false self) induces a psychotic process, particularly the longer it is maintained and the more the true self suffers from the incongruence. Laing describes this process: "The individual's apparently normal and successful adjustment and adaptation to ordinary living is coming to be conceived by his 'true' self as a more and more shameful or ridiculous pretense. If the 'self' [. . .] now conceives the desire to escape . . . and let itself be known without equivocation, one may be witness to the onset of an acute psychosis" (p. 147). The individual who appears to have "gone mad" is simply no longer content to stay shrouded in an internal world where the true self is both silent and invisible. Moreover, in keeping the true self locked away and silent, the individual also may feel complicit in a system that is invalidating and oppressive. In an unknowing nod to what would later be termed "intersectionality," Laing notes that one cannot understand this individual's experience or onset of madness from anyone but the individual herself. That is, from the outside, the experience will be misunderstood, not make sense, or become absent of crucial details due to assumptions of sameness between observer and actor sharing the reality of the false-self system. Laing concludes, "only when one is able to gather from the individual himself the history of his *self*, and *not what a psychiatric history in these circumstances usually is, the history of the false-self system*, that his psychosis becomes explicable" (p. 147).

Laing argues that in order to understand what we call "madness," the history that must be explored and understood is that of the obfuscated true self, not the false self. And, the only person who can give an accounting of the true self's history is the madwoman herself. Therefore, using Laing's ideas, our goal should not be to understand the madwoman from the reader's perspective but rather to consider her point of view as not impaired but legitimate.

One who listens to the madwoman's story from this perspective will be able to recognize that the madwoman will necessarily sound and/or look somewhat crazy if previously she had been going to lengths to conform to her system. To be heard, the madwoman must speak in her true voice in the context of the societal system that does not hear her truth; the reader must bear witness to the madwoman's truth *and* her society's erasure of her. It is only in this listening that a reader can begin to take the madwoman's experience into consciousness.

Being taken into the consciousness of another is different than being momentarily visible. Madwomen often are able to command attention for a moment but they are also easily dismissed. An alternate way of reading the madwoman is to make it a two-person process; it is a dialectic. The madwoman tells us her story, asks us to bear witness to her truth and the false-self system in which she feels trapped. Her story requires someone outside the system to see its entirety clearly. A reader does not need to explain the madwoman's purpose or actions, she needs to recognize her story, direct others to her story, and perhaps, relate to the madwoman's story. In this recognition and sharing of personal narrative, the past is integrated instead of compartmentalized, a dialogue is created, and the false-self system is dismantled both at the level of the individual and at the level of society.

RECOGNITION SCENES

A second idea for consideration is what Northrop Frye calls a "recognition scene." In *Anatomy of Criticism*, Frye (1973) writes: "The culture of the past is not only the memory of mankind, but our own buried life. Study of it leads to a recognition scene, a discovery in which we see, not our past lives, but the total cultural form of our present life" (p. 346). Frye argues that we can only know our current lives by recognizing the past as not only history but also part of the present day. We must see it, not as a history that is outside of us but *in* us as well. The recognition of the past as an irrevocable part of the present is often very painful. It is easy to imagine that one would want to look away, to deny the past, to keep our eyes closed to the false-self system. The challenge in reading the madwoman is to face her fully, to listen to her story, to witness her marginalization without looking away, and to recognize the importance of her story standing in its own right. In sharing the madwoman's story, readers provide a history that may serve as a catalyst for those hearing the story to experience their own recognition scene, to see the ways in which truth can sound "crazy" within their own lives.

MANSPLAINING

A third point in approaching female characters who present as madwomen is more a note about what to resist. In Rebecca Solnit's essay, "Men Explain Things to Me," she details the experience of having men explain things to her, presupposing that, because she is a woman, she does not know much about the subject at hand. The most egregious examples are when men attempt to explain things to her on which she herself is an expert. The essay struck a cultural chord, seemingly speaking to an experience known by many women from various walks of life, who related to the extreme anger and frustration Solnit described feeling when a man condescends to her in this way. Solnit's essay is often credited for inspiring the term "mansplaining," which not only involves men speaking condescendingly to women regarding subjects about which they are well informed but also particularly describes the habit of men explaining things to women that are specific to the experience of being a woman. For example, a man might explain to a woman why she is really upset when a man tells her to "calm down," as if he could understand better than she what is happening in that moment, often dismissing the sexism and gas-lighting many women experience when being told to "calm down" by a man. A related term now also exists, whitesplaining, which describes when Caucasian people speak condescendingly to people of color about issues related to oppression and marginalization. While what happens when readers and critics approach female characters who appear "crazy" is not always or exactly mansplaining or whitesplaining, it is a close cousin. Often, rather than simply using the character's words to illustrate her point, readers will say, "What she means to say is…" or "She's saying this because…" instead of respecting what she has said and trusting that it can speak for itself. To this end, and related to the ideas of the Laing's true self and Frye's recognition scene, I argue that to understand why the madwoman continues to appear, we must first listen to what she is saying and master that. Too often, her voice is immediately lost in our efforts to "explain" her, when perhaps it is she who can explain herself best, and readers need only to recognize her.

STEPPING INTO MADNESS

The madwoman speaks in order to be heard—both by herself and her readers. They must bear witness to her in order for her voice *and* marginalization to be heard and felt. The madwoman seeks not for us to tell her who she is, but rather for us to hear her and witness her invisibility both before and after madness. She is fluent in her second language, that of the false system, though there are some things for which there are no translation from her native, true tongue. She cannot be heard within her own false system; she can only be heard by the reader, who is outside the system. The madwoman craves a scene of recognition.

Each madwoman invites us into conversation, asking us to tolerate hearing her struggle and her negotiations of feeling silenced, invisible, false, or mad. She asks us to bear witness to her truth and marginalization, and from that place, she hopes we might be inspired to share her story and, perhaps, share our own. From this space there can be recognition; the invisible can be seen, the voiceless can be heard, we can have contact with the Other, see the past in our present, mourn what was lost but also recognize that only in telling our stories honestly will we create possibilities for ourselves and our futures. In her mess and craziness, each madwoman invites a reader to turn away or to turn toward. In turning toward the madwoman, a reader sees the madwoman's initial denial of her own true self as she tries to conform, and she also sees that when the madwoman speaks as her true self, she is then denied by others.

The madwoman asks us to bear witness, an act that is not passive and requires both unflinching honesty and courage. Just as psychoanalysis suggests that for therapists to truly understand a patient, they must look within themselves and acknowledge what is stirred, the madwoman does not ask us to analyze her at the exclusion of ourselves. While it may be tempting to read her exclusively as a trope or mirror, the madwoman offers much more: she holds up a two-way mirror, allowing us to see into her as she sees into us, reflecting back parts that we can only see by understanding how we, too, are situated as we relate to others.

APPLICATION: CAN WE LISTEN?

Writers such as Gilbert and Gubar may have focused on the madwoman of the nineteenth century but the madwoman dates back as far as 431 B.C. with the titular character in Euripides's *Medea* and continues into the twentieth century with Sethe in Toni Morrison's *Beloved*. If we think about so-called "psychotic" or delusional symptoms, we understand that the person, in some way, is attempting to rearrange reality so as to be able to cope better. While psychotic reactions often lead to behavior that may seem bizarre, to the person experiencing the delusion, what they see and the actions they take may be a more organized version of the world than was previously known. However, because her words or actions of "madness" are so threatening and foreign to the system, the distress and erasure she wishes to reveal is dismissed. Thus, the madwoman must rely on a reader to be truly seen and heard. Her story is not a form of protest; it is not a selfless act of martyrdom. Instead it is selfish in the truest sense of the word; her madness is the only way she can find absolution from herself, for herself. If we choose to take in her story, it may awaken in us an opportunity to be true to ourselves, not for the sake of society, or women, or our children but, selfishly, for our true selves.

ANDREA YATES

Like novels to the nineteenth century, the news and how it is presented to us as an audience is without a doubt another kind of storytelling. On June 20, 2001, Andrea Yates saw her husband off to work, fed her children breakfast, and then drowned each of her children. She later stated that following their deaths, she immediately made two calls: one to 911 reporting her crime and the other to her husband, asking him to come home. Yates explained her actions stating that she had been possessed by Satan and believed that by killing her children, they would be safe from her influence. Moreover, she believed that when she died via the death penalty, Satan would die with her.[2]

Yates's case captivated the public. There was no doubt that she was "crazy"—there is no act like filicide that best demonstrates craziness in a woman. It is beyond comprehension for most people that a mother could ever even *think* of killing her own children. However, the fact that this act is rendered so unthinkable, so monstrous reveals part of the problem. For the truth is, as any mother who has been driven to her own breaking point might quietly confess, it is, albeit shamefully, not beyond imagination. Anna Quindlen, who felt great sympathy for Yates, interviewed a number of women about the crime. About those interviews she wrote, "[Each woman] has the same reaction. She's appalled; she's aghast. And then she gets this look. And the look says that on some forbidden level she understands" (2001, p 64). Filicide arouses deep discomfort in many women because it challenges the preferred fantasy of the limitless capacity of a mother. In the example of a woman who kills her child, we see the facile conflation of madness and evil in women. A woman who kills her child cannot only be mad, she must also be evil; often her madness is construed as revealing an inherent evil evidenced in the corruption of her maternity, demonstrated by her ability to take her children's lives.

Yates had a history of postpartum depression, hospitalizations, and multiple suicide attempts. As Rebecca Hyman (2004) writes in her article, "Medea of Suburbia: Andrea Yates, Maternal Infanticide, and the Insanity Defense," mental health advocates, feminists, and conservatives all saw in Yates a case in which an example could be made. Mental health advocates pointed to Yates's long history of mental illness, stretching over two years prior to the killings. She had been diagnosed with postpartum depression, had been advised against having further children after her fourth, and had been seen and released from the hospital two days prior to the murder. She was discharged without medication and left to resume full-time care of her children while actively psychotic. Hyman quotes then-president of the National Organization for Women (NOW), Kim Gandy, who noted that Yates's case not only highlighted the challenges many under-resourced women face in motherhood, but also the lack of attention to mental health care nationally, particularly conditions like postpartum psychosis.

Of course, at the time that Yates committed the crime, postpartum depression—let alone postpartum psychosis—was not yet even recognized in the *Diagnostic and Statistical Manual (DSM).*[3] Without a description in the *DSM* and with Texas law stating that a person can only be found not guilty by reason of insanity if the defendant convincingly demonstrates that she cannot differentiate between right and wrong, Yates was perceived as mentally ill *and* criminally and intellectually responsible for her crimes. Here is one of the ways in which Western society grapples with psychosis—by imagining it as a binary of sanity versus insanity. And yet, as anyone who has ever worked with patients experiencing psychosis knows, this is far from the case. Part of the anguish of the illness, particularly when mood dependent, are the ways that delusions and hallucinations are interwoven with an experience that the world itself has gone crazy. Likewise, many people experiencing psychosis have moments of realization in which they are aware that they are not sure which version of reality to trust. Psychosis does *not* mean that one loses her mind; rather, it means one can no longer trust her mind. The system of beliefs often developed within a psychotic state can be experienced as both "wrong" or even "evil" *and* simultaneously necessary, pious, or justified.

Despite being suicidal, diagnosed with postpartum depression, acutely psychotic, and advised not to have more children, Andrea Yates still felt a pressure to be a good woman, which, in her religious belief system meant continuing to have children and caring for them without additional help or resources. While we might feel incredulous or frustrated with Yates's determination to resume these responsibilities in light of her difficulties, we might also wonder about the relative failures of the systems in her life: medical, mental health, family, sociocultural, and religious, all of which believed against all odds, that with enough effort and determination, Yates could somehow withstand the demands of her life and reported symptoms and be a "good mother." Yates's case demonstrated the resistance of the false-self system to hearing one's true self, as many people continued to judge her as competent despite her showing that she was falling apart. Consider that, although she was taken to the hospital two days before the murders, Yates was evaluated and judged fit to resume her caretaking responsibilities.

Yates's story, and our collective responses to her story, connect deeply with the madwoman figured in literature. It is not the madwoman alone who is mad, but the society in which she lives. Part of that madness is a shared, systemic delusion about women, that despite all odds and challenges, all injuries and mental anguish, women and especially women who have become mothers, are not expected to break. When it comes to their roles as caregivers, women are often expected to be limitless resources, responding with grace and patience no matter how overwhelming external and internal stressors become. It is their obligation as women and as mothers to be not only self-sacrificing but even masochistic at times. It is as if, when a woman becomes a mother, she forfeits her humanity—the vulnerability that might cause her to succumb to the pressures inside and outside of her. To imagine that all women are capable of willing themselves to withstand any pain they face for the sake of their children is delusional. Other women have a particular obligation to speak up and challenge this delusion. Instead of feigning incredulity, we must acknowledge the unattainable expectations. Rather than using denial to pretend that this only happens to "other" women, we must be vocal that some combination of privilege and grace only it makes her and not us.

MEDEA

It is no accident that Hyman (2004) refers to Andrea Yates as the "Modern Medea." Perhaps the earliest example of a literary madwoman, Medea's story has enthralled readers for thousands of years. In Euripides's version, which is the most widely-read, Medea is presented as a figure of striking contrasts. Descended from gods, highly intelligent, and uncommonly persuasive, Medea is a woman unlike any other; with the favor of the gods, the skill of a sorceress, and the cunning of a man, Medea goes after what she wants, taking things without apology or shame. She is such a powerful figure that, even within the play, it is she who is largely seen as responsible for Jason's success in acquiring the Golden Fleece, a feat that would have been impossible without her calculation, skill, and fratricide.

It is clear from the beginning of the play that the only thing Medea wants is for Jason to love her, marry her, and take her away from Colchis. She locates her acceptance and freedom in him. Thus, when Jason abandons her for Glauce, it is a mistake to read her as merely a "jilted lover." Medea's rage is not one of merely jealousy but abandonment and realization that all of her sacrifices have been for naught. Despite intellectually realizing she is superior to him in a variety of ways, emotionally she has wanted only his love and allegiance. When he takes this away, her world is thrown into total chaos and her choices no longer makes sense. The impossibility of continuing in the false-system she has tried to inhabit in exchange for Jason's love is shattered. Wild with grief and anger, Medea's world collapses and she goes mad, killing Glauce and then her own children. These two acts are now the only things that make sense in her world, the only two ways she can see to touch Jason's heart and protect her children. The evidence that her actions are seen as a conflation between madness and evil are supported by the Chorus's reaction to her children's death sand their description of her as "evil" (see lines 1406–1411).

In the 1960s, many Classical scholars revisited *Medea* and saw her as a victim of patriarchy, replacing reading her as evil to seeing her as a mistreated woman made "mad" by her own jealousy and despair. But Medea is railing against far more than mistreatment by a single person. In Eleanor Wilner's 1998 translation of *Medea*, which she completed with the help of Inés Azar, Wilner reflected on her own understanding of the titular madwoman; she compared her own experience of teaching the play in the 1960s and 1970s with her efforts to translate the play on the cusp of the twenty-first century. Wilner (1998) recalls that "the earlier Medea, the character, . . . was a figure for the betrayed woman and proto-feminist, the superior alien" (p. 3). And certainly, this was the version of the play that I was taught even in the mid-1990s.

At the time of my own first reading of *Medea*, I remember the uneasy feeling I had. On the one hand, I felt gratified to hear Medea's actions contextualized. Certainly it was not hard to see the way Jason had used her for his own gain and then discarded her, but it also felt reductive to take strong and exceptional woman presented and read her as suddenly broken by jealous. I was simultaneously taking a Great Novels course, reading *Anna Karenina*, *Madame Bovary*, *The House of Mirth*, *The Awakening*, *Rabbit, Run*, and *them*, among others. The synergy of reading these novels alongside *Medea* left me wondering what it was that, regardless of time and place, many women seemed destined to lives with such acute suffering and fits of "madness" that death was often preferable to living.

As Wilner reflects on her discoveries while translating the text, she, too, expresses a similar discomfort with this facile understanding of Medea. As she tries to understand her former reading of the text with the one she finds herself translating, she observes something missed on her earlier readings: "The Chorus, Jason, Creon, and Medea all mouth pieties their actions or their next speech belie. The difference between Medea and the other characters in this regard is that she is aware of her (and their) duplicity, and uses that awareness to manipulate others" (p. 4). Wilner uses this to explore the power differential between Medea and Jason; she sees Medea possessing the "innate" power and Jason possessing the "institutional" power, and she rightly draws attention to the stress that such an inherent power imbalance would create.

But, it was not the difference in power that was Medea's undoing. Medea lives in a world where she *sees through the veil*, both for herself and others; in seeing the duplicity of herself and others, she is already teetering dangerously on a high-wire of attempting to straddle what Laing might call the false-self and true-self systems. She is living with a tremendous cognitive dissonance, seeing clearly her duplicity and that of others, but operating in the world by colluding, by treating others as though they are the pious beings they present themselves to be. It is only through her madness, her act of killing her children, that the Chorus, and we as readers, are thrust into Medea's subjectivity and forced to confront this in ourselves. Wilner captures this as she contemplates:

> We are left to . . . face without consolation the atrocious acts that people, when the usual restraints fall away, are capable of committing . . . And the complicity of the on-stage audience does raise questions about that other audience, over two millennia old now, of which we are a part (p. 11).

Of course, one might push against the atrociousness that Wilner situates in Medea herself, and instead see it as the inevitable collateral of a system that asks a woman to live knowing and seeing one truth in herself while living a socially constructed and reinforced lie that demeans her. It is Medea's realization that to go on living in this world means not only the death of her own soul but the death of her children's. It is her refusal to bear the responsibility for her children being spiritually killed that leads to her belief that the only choice available to her is to kill her children herself. Medea considers that death by another hand would truly be a murder and "cruel," so she cries out, "Since they must die in any case, / then let me, who gave them birth, be the bearer / of their death. Heart, put on your armor now!" (lines 1347–1349).

SETHE

From Medea, the modern reader may recognize Sethe's dilemma in Tony Morrison's *Beloved*. The novel focuses primarily on Sethe's life after her decision to kill her infant daughter rather than allow her to be taken from her into slavery. Following what can best be described as a mammary rape (two white men steal her breast milk), Sethe is reeling from being unable to assert autonomy over her own body; she attempts to assert her own agency in the only way she can see how, killing her daughter rather than allowing her to be dirtied by slavery in the way she has been. This action occurs very early in the narrative, and the majority of the novel focuses on Sethe's attempt to live with this act and to make sense of it for herself, even as she continues to see and hear her infant daughter as a ghost of sorts. While *Medea* shows us the lead up to the collapse of the false self, *Beloved* shows us the aftermath, the shattering that occurs when the madwoman's true self emerges and she cannot return to living as her false self.

Sethe, as a young slave, has an idea of herself as a person that does not correspond with her social status, much like Medea, a woman of the gods living as a mortal. Sethe sees herself as human but lives among those who see her as chattel. Sethe perceives her body as her own but this is not true under slavery. Like Medea learning about her own vulnerability when she is cast aside by Jason, Sethe realizes there is no escaping how she is seen when Schoolteacher's nephews (white men) steal her breastmilk.

In the act of the mammary rape is the argument that her body is not her own. The fact that her milk is stolen complicates matters, as it suggests that not only is Sethe helpless to assert autonomy over her own body but also she is powerless to protect her child as she cannot even keep her breastmilk safe to feed her daughter. The greatest sin of slavery is its dehumanization—its ability to take a person and tell her that her body is not her own and that she has no say in how it will be seen or touched. This is articulated as Sethe recalls Paul D's departure:

> That anybody white could take your whole self for anything that came to mind. Not just work, kill, or maim you, but dirty you. Dirty you so bad you couldn't like yourself anymore. (p. 295)

Sethe experiences the mammary rape as a kind of death, and it is in this moment that her madness takes root; she can no longer straddle the false-self and true-self worlds. She reflects, "And though she and others lived through and got over it, she could never let it happen to her own. The best thing she was, was her children" (p. 295). It is this moment of recognition that leads her to behead Beloved, and it remains understood as a moment of madness because, as the narration of *Beloved* reveals, Sethe tries to put this moment of recognition out of her mind by forgetting the past in order to return to the false-self world. Because she cannot see her own way out of the system she is in, she forgets her truth and instead regards herself as mad. The text makes repeated references to Sethe's daily work of "beating back the past" (p. 86), and looking for ways to distract herself from "remembering something she had forgotten she knew" (p. 73).

Using Laing's theory (1960), killing Beloved reveals Sethe's true self's "desire to escape from shut-upness" (p. 147). Following the mammary rape and seeing that her own daughter is now at risk, she can no longer bear to act within the false-self system. When Sethe takes the handsaw to Beloved's neck, she is acting out of self-preservation—she loves her children but, as her own reflection reveals, she also has transferred her sense of self and worthiness that slavery has taken from her to her children. She has not accepted what has happened to her but has instead transferred her desire for remaining human and unsullied to her children, and she sees killing Beloved as the only way to not only save her child but to save herself.

This demonstrates how the violation of her children being enslaved by Schoolteacher would be doubly devastating to Sethe, much as Medea imagines the abandonment of her children at the hands of Jason and as Andrea Yates envisioned her children's corruption by Satan. Their situations are unique and their contexts vastly different, but perhaps across these varied contexts what can be understood about madness in women, particularly as it is often portrayed in literature or even as it is covered in media, is that being complicit in subjecting one's offspring to the same limbo between false self and true is intolerable; that sometimes, given an impossible choice, madness ensues as a mother tries to contemplate which is worse: a physical death or a psychic/emotional one. Most startlingly, in that moment, these women wrestle with the knowledge that the only way to protect not only their children but also their own true selves is to act in the only way they can imagine that could to spare their children the same fate.

What Sethe does not see until the end of the novel is that Schoolteacher's nephews did not take all she had. They have horribly violated her but the very fact that she still fights the helplessness represented in Schoolteacher suggests that she has not relinquished her own sense of agency. Killing Beloved is wrong but, by the end of the novel, we understand that what haunts Sethe is not the fact that she killed Beloved but the knowledge that she killed Beloved partly out of a desire to not only "save" Beloved but also to save what was left of herself.

Sethe has survived slavery but she is plagued with survivor's guilt, particularly as she still splits her identity and projects those qualities she sees as worthy onto her children. The debt Sethe owes at the end of the novel is not to Beloved. Sethe must forgive herself for saving herself in the act of sacrificing her daughter, who she saw as the embodiment of her own goodness. When she can finally recognize, in Paul D's words, that she is her "own best thing" (p. 322), she has finally achieved that which can allow her madness to remit: she has integrated the past into the present and stepped out of the false-self system. Sethe accepts the death of Beloved as part of who she is, for at least a moment, and in that space, she no longer sees and hears Beloved;

Sethe's fate after the narrative of the novel largely depends on whether or not she can hold onto her past as part of who she is in the future.

CONCLUSION

By reading Sethe's "mad" act of killing Beloved in this way, we better understand the repeated sentence at the end of the novel, "It was not a story to pass on," and "This was not a story to pass on" (p. 323–24). In its first iteration, Sethe must know and accept her history in order to free herself from the intergenerational trauma that maintains its power in its unspeakableness. She must know and remember that which she tries to forget. In its second utterance, we understand the emphasis now means that once Sethe knows the story and has claimed it, she must realize it is not a story to be reenacted. Once the act is understood, its effects must remain as a part of her present, always, in order to stop it from happening again, to step out of the false-self system and to remain in touch with her truth, even if painful. In its final repetition, the reader sees that the sentence is applied to she herself. As Sethe must know the story, so, too, must we. It is not a story for us to deny or repeat; we must bear witness to it. If we do not want our children to inherit this unspoken burden, then we must accept responsibility for our cultural history and we must acknowledge its part in our present. We must not try to "understand" how or why Sethe came to take Beloved's life but recognize her "madness" and the action she took as a moment of radical departure from the false-self system in which she had been living; we must recognize and give voice to the false-self system in which we all try to live while denying our true selves. It is not a story to pass on, but it is a story that will be passed on without that recognition, without the awakening at the level of the system.

This is the allure of the madwoman in literature. She is the canary in the coal mine. Each woman's story is her own; each one's suffering and particular madness unique. She is not a stand-in for the author and she does not carry a universal message. Each woman reveals her own incredibly personal and painful history of what it is to be unknown, unseen, and trapped in a system that asks you to be someone you are not and can never be. While vastly different, these female characters reveal a struggle that has spanned thousands of years. As long as hierarchies of gender, race, sexuality, and class exists, and as long women continue to feel confined in systems that require the surrender of so much of their true selves, madwomen will continue to be seen in our stories. We must bear witness to their unique stories and share their words, their individual experiences of marginalization.

The examples of madwomen discussed here display a particular kind of madness, the kind humanity most fears, which is the killing of one's offspring in an attempt to save both the children and the women themselves. As these women come to see that their sacrifice of their true self will not protect their children from their same fate of oppression, the madwomen will take the only action left: they will leave the false self behind and inhabit a place that is true and yet mad—both in its sudden departure from previous behavior and its desperation. These women seek to claim space and voices for themselves and their children by taking their children's lives rather than being complicit in their children's subjugation. There is no essential truth to be taken from the madwomen in literature, but there are truths to be heard and felt, unique to each woman.

REFERENCES

Charatan, F., Eaton, F., & Eaton, L. (2002). Woman may face death penalty in postnatal depression case. *BMJ : British Medical Journal, 324*(7338), 634.

Chester, P. (1972). *Women and Madness* Garden City, NY: Doubleday,

Chödrön, P. (2000). *When Things Fall Apart: Heart Advice for Difficult Times.* Boston: Shambhala.

Euripedes. (1998). *Medea.* (E. Wilner, Trans.) Philadelphia: University of Pennsylvania Press.

Frye, N. (1973) *Anatomy of Criticism: Four Essays.* Princeton: Princeton University Press.

Gilbert, S. & Gubar, S. (1979). *The Madwoman in the Attic: The Woman Writer and the Nineteenth-century Literary Imagination.* New Haven, CT: Yale University Press.

Hyman, R. (2004). Medea of Suburbia: Andrea Yates, Maternal Infanticide, and the Insanity Defense. *Women's Studies Quarterly, 32*, 192–210.

Laing, R. D. (1960). *The Divided Self.* New York: Pantheon Books.

Lorde, A. (1984). *Sister Outsider: Essays and Speeches*. Trumansburg, NY: Crossing Press.

Morrison, T. *Beloved*. New York: Columbia University Press.

Quindlen, A. (2001, February 7). Playing God on no sleep. *Newsweek*, 64.

Read, J. & Dillon, J. (2013). *Models of Madness: Psychological, Social, and Biological Approaches to Psychosis.* New York: Routledge.

Schlichter, A. (2003). Critical Madness, Enunciative Excess: The Figure of the Madwoman in Postmodern Feminist Texts. *Cultural Studies, Critical Methodologies, 3* (3) 308–29.

Solnit, R. (2014). *Men Explain Things to Me.* Chicago: Haymarket Books.

Solnit, R. (2017). *The Mother of All Questions*. Chicago: Haymarket Books.

Wilner, E. (1998). *Translator's Preface to Medea.*. Philadelphia: University of Pennsylvania Press.

NOTES

1. Disability studies began as an academic discipline in the mid-1980s and began to gain academic visibility in the United States in the mid-1990s, both well after the publication of Gilbert and Gubar's work. Disability studies has encouraged readers and critics to think about the way in which physical and mental disabilities are yet another social construct, with medical models frequently unfairly stigmatizing persons who present with physical and mental difference as impaired and "other." Within the critique of both disability studies and mental health advocacy exists the continuing question of the extent to which criteria for mental illnesses are characteristics seemingly attributed more predominantly to women, or are outgrowths of trauma, which women of most cultures face in greater proportion than men. So as will be discussed more in the next section, one might also wonder about how even the medical and psychological classifications of illnesses typical of psychosis are defined in such a way as to necessarily diagnose more women than men.

2. See Charatan, F., Eaton, F., & Eaton, L. (2002). Woman may face death penalty in postnatal depression case. *BMJ : British Medical Journal, 324*(7338), 634.

3. In 2013, the *DSM-V* finally included language to describe postpartum depression, though many would argue it is still not as inclusive or helpful as it could be. Of note in particular to this case, *DSM-V* does state that the chance of postpartum psychosis increases with subsequent pregnancies following episodes of postpartum depression.

Chapter Three

Stories

Berta Britz

I hear, see, and sense what others around me don't. Sometimes my beliefs and thoughts are anomalous. Diagnosed with psychosis in adolescence, I lived with limiting beliefs about my experiences for over forty years—these were beliefs that I personally generated and that were also taught and imposed on me by others. My growth depended on overcoming my passivity, as I swallowed my emotions throughout infancy, childhood, adolescence, and adulthood. It is not easy to differentiate "negative symptoms" of psychosis from the passivity, helplessness, and hopelessness reinforced in our cultural institutions—family, schools and hospitals. As I moved through roles of damaged child, chronic institutionalized patient, worker, student, and disabled worker, to person, I forged connections and re-discovered a healthy sexuality. In this chapter I describe my process of becoming human, my movement toward wholeness. I will use stories to highlight the impact of gender, culture, and context across generations. They are stories about my relationship to "the other," stories about the meaning I made of "the other" in me, in family and in culture, and the meaning I made of "the other" outside me. They are stories of movement from a binary vision of myself and others that reflected dominant family/societal/cultural presuppositions about ethics, health, disease, gender, sex roles, sexual orientations, politics, and power, to a dynamic and inclusive acceptance of self and co-creation of self in relation to "other" from a "both/and" perspective.

Telling our own stories allows us to know ourselves differently, to become more fully ourselves in a liberating wholeness. We are a multi-dimensional weaving of many-colored threads that includes the space between words, between people, between breaths. Telling our stories helps bring harmony from the diverse languages of dissonance, discord, varied tempos, depth, and scope through the co-creating of meanings within relationships. As Audre Lorde wrote, "If I didn't define myself for myself, I would be crunched into other people's fantasies for me and eaten alive" (Lorde, 1982, p. 134). If my story isn't spoken and heard, it is closed—fossilized. I have traversed a labyrinthine path to discovery, and discovered ways of "knowing" differently. This layered process of exploration led me back to my source, my center, my soul. In T. S. Eliot's words, I returned to "know the place for the first time" (Eliot, 1952, p.145).

My memories of times when I experienced vulnerability are solid, sunk deep. They root me in soil fertilized by others—ancestors, family, animals, trees, friends, and strangers, held by all I've experienced with those I have known and been known by, and our shared stories of her/history, myth, poetry, music, religion. My drive to discover and learn has carried me through chaos, pain, confusion, and loss. My journey has been fueled by relationships. While some relationships co-created paths of meaning with me, others blocked or eroded the paths.

I grew up with fear dominating my life. I was so terrified that I lived life as a victim. It was hard to learn in school and, because my fear confused me, I was perceived as developmentally delayed and out of sync with my peers. I lacked trust and remained mostly silent, mostly alone, intent on hiding the secret of my vulnerabilities and holding loyalty to others. The people I depended on did and said things that harmed as well as helped me and, even though we loved each other, I don't think they were aware of my experience. I survived in separate, sometimes parallel, sometimes overlapping, worlds. My early life was a secret search to figure out what was real and true, because it was often unclear to me what was truly outside me or inside me.

I had three primary caregivers: my mother, my brother, and the lady who was paid to babysit, cook, and clean when my mother was at work and my brother was in school. She was loving and gentle, soothingly French Canadian—her personal lyrics and melody composed from notes and tempo syncopated by family tragedies, conflicts, and painful moods not spoken.

My mother was a strong woman at a time when our society did not encourage strong women. Born in 1913, she graduated from college and managed a business. She idealized her mother, Bertha, who transcended the usual female roles of her day. Although my grandmother died while I was still in utero, my given name was derived from her name, and she was a palpable presence in my early years. I believed she observed me and everything I did, and I often begged for her forgiveness for my perceived badness. At the same time, although I felt that if anyone could see me and still accept me, it was this grandmother, I sometimes doubted that even she could forgive my badness.

Memory carries truth even when evidence is unclear. One of my earliest memories was infant-me in the crib in our first house, feeling a gurgling oneness, my diaper full, and a torso bent over with an arm reaching toward me. A sweet melodic voice, emitting from an odor of perfumed powder, asked what I had done. Sweet and bitter combined. Mixed messages absorbed.

I learned from stories I picked up from people around me, including the perceptions I now name "voices." I assumed that the family, caregivers, teachers, and rabbis who preceded me knew and understood what I didn't. I was scared. Nothing made sense to me, so I spent my childhood and youth secretly seeking and trying to digest all clues. It was not safe to acknowledge not-knowing or my terror, because I saw everyone as taller and smarter and stronger than I.

During my childhood I hid my vulnerability, did not acknowledge my disconnection or my needs. My language was action and absence. As an adolescent and adult, my disconnection was palpable. My language and thoughts were not understood by others. Verbalization didn't work. I spoke little and when I did speak or write, it was mixed up, not understood by others. Words meant different things to me. I didn't speak directly—my thoughts and beliefs were dangerous, embodied in terrorizing voices. I connected in code with the people I encountered, and my voices used their own codes to both command and obfuscate.

My mother told me the story of my birth and babyhood during special private times. The stories carried her own particular vocabulary for telling and her own unique lens for seeing. She was my story's first author. I began on Halloween 1950. She saw the size of my foot and worried that she had given birth to a monster. Then was shown that she was looking through a magnifying glass.

Mommy told me how voracious a baby I was when she tried to breast-feed. I hurt her nipples so much that she almost resorted to bottle feeding. She believed that breastfeeding was "right," so she persevered and received a salve from her doctor. For my mother God was her conscience, so doing "right" was divine imperative.

My mother conveyed her devastation at the loss of her own mother, whose death left her facing huge demands for life skills she had never acquired. Mother's sense of inadequacy and rage in relation to our family was embodied in her frustrated attempts to assume traditionally female roles of cook, baker, caregiver to baby-me, while the identity and competence she experienced and valued was traditionally male.

She also told me about giving me baths, explaining that it was "right" and important to her that she bathe infant-me. She didn't want to allow others to take on that responsibility and "pleasure." She told me about washing and gently splashing me in the bath until she got carried away and held my head under the water till my breath was almost gone. I grew up afraid of water and carrying the weight of having survived.

My mother dominated my father and managed our family household, as well as doing bookkeeping for my father's law practice and co-managing the meat packing plant she and her sole surviving brother inherited from their parents. Having lived through the Great Depression, my parents never lost their fear of scarcity. My father's experience of immigrant poverty and his own father's apparent but unspeakable undependability seemed to ignite a drive to prove his "manhood" to provide financially for our family with as little input from my mother's income as possible. We were Jewish in a predominantly Christian community and, to me, we seemed different and separate from most Jewish people as well. My parents carried a sense of insecurity and an identity of being "socially less-than" that seemed to propel their determination to both assimilate and stay separate from our communities. My father's family had fled pogroms in Russia to settle in the United Kingdom, and he was brought to the United States from Wales as a boy. I heard stories from an early age about the Nazi Holocaust and my father's inability to secure the release and emigration of my mother's relatives from Poland and Germany. I struggled to understand my place in an unsafe large world that included our unsafe, smaller family world.

With the best of intentions, my mother began trying to toilet train me at six-months of age but, even at ten years old, I still wet the bed on occasion. I have no memory of this beginning, but retain the image from the photo of me strapped to a toilet with a leather belt. I do recall, in grueling detail, my long struggle to wake with dry sheets. It was most often my brother's job to change my diapers. Since I wore them for so long, he taught my sister to help. She wasn't strong or tall enough, so he told me to lie on the floor and instructed me to lift my bottom by saying, "Up girl." He was my hero.

He also stimulated himself and me sexually. I didn't understand what that meant. During my childhood, I felt sexually aroused a lot and it contributed to my sense of core badness. My parents were unaware of my brother's sexual behavior and depended on him as a key babysitter and childcare provider. I imagine that he felt lonely and overwhelmed after our maternal grandmother died. My mother's story of him was that he had exceptional brilliance and an amazing sense of direction from toddlerhood. It was his role to lead, guide, and teach—even before he was school-age—and I learned from him. My experience of helplessness, combined with his exceptional power, emerged from my mother's stories about both my brother and me. My mother and brother were the gods I worshipped.

Mommy took me into the bathroom with her when she used the toilet. I remember the times when she wiped herself and showed me the toilet paper with mucus on it. She said, "See what you've done to me!" She told me that my badness was harming her. I watched her douche, with no understanding of what it was. I learned that I was poisoning her. I tried not to cause harm but continually made mistakes and misbehaved, and she taught me that I caused bad things to happen in the world.

Stories and books provided the foundation for my search to make sense of the world. I gathered all clues from outside to try to populate my inside understanding. One of my guides was "Hop-O'- My-Thumb," a story of how the youngest and smallest of seven children whose parents repeatedly abandoned them in the forest, was able to save himself, his siblings, and eventually his parents, King and country. I memorized many of the stories and verses that others read to me. I pretended to read by reciting them, so many people assumed that I knew much that actually mystified me and I conspired to preserve my/our secrets.

I had ongoing nightmares where I frantically tried to escape from enemies. I ran and ran until finally, giving up, I surrendered and fell fast. I fell and fell and fell but, when I hit the ground, I landed gently and woke. Other times, I dreamed that my mother was in danger and I was the only one present to save her. I tried to drive her to the hospital but my legs were far too short to reach the gas or brake pedals. I couldn't keep her alive. I wasn't enough.

In second grade I was placed in a special class. In those days, our public school had no "special education," only a speech therapist for someone whose speech was hard to understand. Then they created our class. My understanding was that I was considered "retarded." It was never explained to me, so "defect" was what I absorbed. My mother and I understood being "different" as being "less-than," which translated to "bad."

Miss Bramble, that second grade teacher, taught me to listen with both my ears and my eyes, to watch a speaker in order to take in the message. I learned to read! That breakthrough opened worlds containing much new evidence in my search for "real and true." I can still taste the triumph I felt on the day I was able to read and pronounce the word, "giraffe." Miss Bramble engaged with me and taught me to attend. "I want to see those dark brown eyes," she would declare. Hers was a powerful gift. Miss Bramble's accepting attitude and presence were primary sources enabling me to use her lessons in my quest for making sense of almost incomprehensible worlds.

My adventures walking and later riding a bike to school were fodder for both fascination and terror. I could not read or tell time. On my journey to school, if it was quiet, with no children visible, I knew that I was either very early or very late. Surprisingly, I was only tardy once. I was in the third grade, and it was on one of those eerily quiet days when I was rushing to get there. I flipped over my bike's handlebars. Bleeding, and worried that I would be sent to the principal's office, I righted myself and pressed forward to class where I collapsed. I woke up in a car on the way to the doctor's.

I was seven, and it was the year my brother went to college. I lost him. His sexual gratification abuse with me ended. I felt abandoned. I continued to

feel extremely sexual though I had no understanding of it. I had an anomalous, never spoken-aloud language and I continued masturbating and holding
and releasing my urine to bring myself pleasure and release. I confused my
belly with an entry to sex based on my experience with my brother. I witnessed an older, beer-soaked male relative perform for me as he urinated, and
it looked like it was arching from his navel. I learned from my mother that
babies grew from seeds planted in a woman's "belly-button." My belief that I
had a tiny penis that no one else knew about was another secret stored deep
in private shame.

I sucked my thumb for my entire childhood and adolescence, stopping in
my late twenties. My parents worked hard to stop my thumb sucking. They
painted my thumb with very bad tasting stuff, lectured, cajoled, punished,
and mocked me. No one could come between me and my thumb. Sucking my
thumb was soothing and significant—it kept me alive.

Animals and trees also preserved me. When I was four, I was sent to day
camp. It was another confusing, overwhelming situation to navigate. They
tried to teach me to swim in a shallow pool. I breathed terror but had no
words to explain. They tried to teach me to make a lanyard from "boondog-
gle," but I couldn't follow directions. The day camp owners had a farm and
invited me to go there with them on a weekend. My parents gave their
permission, and I never returned to day camp. That was the beginning of my
connecting with caring people outside the orbit of family and religious
school. I found refuge in animals and nature, and in the adults who taught me
important life lessons. I learned how to hold a fork for eating, how to share
simple fun and chores. I learned to take care of animals and our environment.
I learned to sing, clap, and play with others, thus building new neural pathways. I learned to take care of and ride horses and eventually to swim in a
lake. I learned to connect with others to help them learn as well. Instead of
blaming and shaming me for my lack of abilities, they taught me. The owners
of the farm became a second family to me. My inclusion deepened after they
were shaken by the death of their older son in a car accident. They nurtured
me in space he had occupied.

Headaches punctured and punctuated my early life. When I was six, a
neurologist diagnosed and treated me for a seizure disorder. Later the diagnosis was changed to migraine headaches. I missed large chunks of school and
opportunities for social connection starting in the fourth grade when I was
nine years old. I spent much of elementary school in my parents' bed watching *I Love Lucy* and *Make Room for Daddy*, often in excruciating pain. As I
writhed, wishing for death and blaming myself for having thrown away my
pills, I felt trapped.

During the summer of 1962, I was at the farm that my "adopted" family
had developed into an overnight camp. I received a letter from my mother
with instructions to destroy it after reading. She wrote that my father had

cancer of the larynx and would be getting treatment for it in Chicago. I was to stay at the farm after camp was over until they came home from Chicago. It was important to keep my father's cancer a secret from everyone outside the family. I panicked that I had caused my father's cancer and assumed he would die from it. My worst guilt was that I didn't think I loved my father and would not experience any real grief and I would be exposed. I wrote a letter to my "adopted" mother, pouring out anguished guilt, painful shame, and apology but failed to sign my name. She assumed that an adult counselor had written it, and I felt crushed that she couldn't recognize my story even without my signature. My lonely secrets stirred me to seek solace from the hills. I climbed to the highest point and looked out over the hills and lakes. As I walked down the hill, I came to a group of several trees whose trunks formed a circle. Two horses stood head-to-tail in the shade, swishing flies away from each other's faces. I climbed into the middle of the tree trunks and hugged them. Bark scraping my arms, I squeezed tight—releasing and taking in natural succor.

When I was in seventh grade, a man whom I knew from horseback riding hanged himself. I looked ill and expressed fatigue in addition to headaches, so my family doctor hospitalized me for tests. My roommate in the hospital had a life-threatening diagnosis, and I was relatively healthy. I felt ashamed for my relative health compared to her likely death and assumed that was the message my doctor intended. The following year, I was in math class when we learned that John F. Kennedy had been shot. I watched my teacher's expression as he learned the news before he told us. He was a kind teacher who had seen me as an individual and had been coaching me to take math tests by shifting my focus to work faster and finish, rather than sinking into one challenging problem. I observed his shock and pain, and I perceived death stalking me.

That year everyone took standardized tests, and expectations for me changed. I felt humiliated in front of my English class when the teacher questioned my high achievement in all subjects except math. That teacher revised her view of my capacity and refused to allow me to continue writing book reports on books I enjoyed like *The Black Stallion* and *Nancy Drew.* So I proposed *Of Human Bondage,* but she found that choice too adult, and we settled on *How Green Was My Valley.* I read *Of Human Bondage* that summer but had no one to dialogue with about its meaning.

In the ninth grade, I was surprised to find myself placed in the advanced English class next to those students who had been tracked together in the familiar elite group throughout their schooling. My alien status didn't change but I was able to read a wonderful translation of Homer's *The Odyssey,* which I would have missed had I stayed with my former cohort. It stimulated my thoughts about courage and journeying home, an exciting, dangerous adventure fueled by commitment, loyalty, and love.

That Christmas vacation, my family visited my mother's cousin in northern California, where I had an appointment with a neurologist. He worked with a psychologist and, upon our arrival, we were informed that I was required to see the psychologist first. The psychologist evaluated me by administering lots of tests and treating me with a warm, cautious respect. I allowed my usual guardedness to lessen, enjoying her manner and the tests which seemed fascinating, and in no way related to my headaches or experiences living in family and school. I offered two or more answers for almost every question asked, reflecting my extreme ambivalence and the pleasure I derived from confiding multiple explanations. This psychologist listened to me for what felt like the first time. This was true for the IQ testing as well as for the projective tests like the Thematic Apperception Test (TAT). Later when the neurologist recommended that I get a psychiatric evaluation, I felt furious and scared—swept up in my perception of the psychologist's betrayal of my relative openness in participating in the testing and panicked that I had carelessly betrayed and endangered myself and my family, especially my mother.

My mother was shocked. Once home, she turned to the family doctor for protection and expert advice. He suggested seeking a psychiatric evaluation but withholding the psychologist's recommendation in order to prevent biasing the psychiatrist. This time I dutifully kept my guard up and answered the psychiatrist's questions with total honesty but without full truth. After my three-session evaluation, the psychiatrist, who knew my father from court and synagogue, reported that he wished more young people were like me and gave no diagnosis.

My parents did their best to parent and they feared exposing the family to outsiders' judgements. I felt we were haunted by Nazi threats even though the war was over for the rest of the world. My parents required me to participate in my religious confirmation ceremony at fourteen, despite my philosophical objection. At sixteen when I proposed sharing an apartment with an older friend, a counselor at the camp where I had been a counselor-in-training, my parents immediately rejected the arrangment as a negative reflection on them. I had couched the proposal carefully, to emphasize ongoing skill building, work, and school, but to no avail.

My parents tried to blend in with the dominant culture, and I felt alienated. My favorite clothes were ragged blue jeans and a faded red checked flannel shirt which had belonged to my brother. My father forbade me to go downtown dressed as myself, looking like an outcast. I did not rebel. I stayed invisible, although I sided with anti-war protesters, civil rights marchers, and also with poor people who rioted. My mother accepted my politics theoretically but she could not see me. I heard about the Vietnamese monks who immolated themselves. I protested silently. I was afraid to speak. I was afraid to see and be seen/known by others. The truth of me was invisible to everyone but animals. When I read Martin Buber's description of his I-Thou relationship with a horse, I resonated. I caught a glimmer of what was possible in relationships. I wrote to the rabbi about my guilt for not loving my dad. The rabbi wrote back that we were commanded to honor our fathers and mothers, not to love them. I was astounded at that distinction, and it was hard to believe.

After escaping the first psychiatric diagnosis, I lived for a year in desperation and despair before my appointment with a new neurologist. This time the neurologist was a man who had gone to elementary school with my mother. During the examination, I told him that he was my second-to-last resort. He asked what my last resort was, and I acknowledged that it was a psychiatrist. He was kind and brave enough to tell my mother that he recommended that she take me to a psychiatrist. Hurt and humiliated, she did as the expert directed. This psychiatrist began, "Have you ever felt down in the dumps? How far?" He seemed like a new lifeline but this line took me to years of institutionalization, to a different type of imprisonment, fossilization and definition by different deities.

He complained that it was like pulling teeth to get me to speak. He prescribed medications and I tried to attend my senior year of high school. Upon returning to school after a long absence, I was scheduled to take a make-up exam for Trigonometry and was anxious. During my economics class prior to the make-up exam, my neck went into hyperextension. It was beyond my control and I didn't understand. It was impossible to bring my head down, even when the teacher tried to manually move it to my desk. I silently berated myself for creating a spectacle just because I was scared to take a math test. Of course, the actual culprit was the Stelazine that had been prescribed. After I was removed from class, taken home, and injected with Benadryl, my head magically returned to its usual posture. My status as a pariah was set in stone.

Around this time, my friend Judy died. We first met on the farm when I was four. She had given me piggy-back rides, taught me to hold a fork, to care for horses, and to swim. Later she taught me to teach and nurture younger children. She was my life preserver. I had attended her wedding to her sweetheart, a man who was then sent to the Vietnam War. Shortly after he returned, she had a heart attack and died. It was incomprehensible. She was young, strong, and athletic. Her heart was vulnerable. My voices bombarded me, and I was lost. My mother took me to the funeral home for the viewing. Judy's body was clothed in her wedding gown, her skin looked like wax. I missed her funeral.

Instead of going to Reed College—the only college I applied to because it was my brother's recommendation—I went to the mental hospital. I missed other important funerals too, the chance to communally grieve and acknowledge my real loss of significant animals and people. I missed anti-war protests and the first walk on the moon. I received a letter from a boyfriend, whom I had met at a camp for Jewish teenagers. Now a student at Kent State University, he described his learning and blossoming into personhood. He asked me to explain what I was doing in the mental hospital. My birthdays passed too.

For a long time, I lived a death-in-life. My belief that I was not human was a belief that endured for decades. It was declared by voices and also confirmed and reflected in the objectifying way I was conceptualized and treated by the psychiatric system. It was the role and responsibility of psychiatric professionals to enact the system's vision to try to fix or at least manage me. Voices intoned, "You belong in flames. Set yourself on fire." They said "All that you touch is tainted." "Stab the eyes, slash the arms." Voice messages echoed and amplified the messages I received as a young child. They preyed on fear and claimed to be all-powerful and all-knowing. Voices intoned my powerlessness. I was afraid of my voices, afraid of myself. Well-intentioned male psychiatrists tried to shut down those voices without ever considering or acknowledging that the messages might mean something to me. They claimed that my experience was not real and required annihilation. The psychiatric system was afraid of my voices, afraid of me. Both my voices and psychiatry agreed: my having choice was dangerous and not to be tolerated. I had swallowed the beliefs of my voices and the assumptions of psychiatry. Whether my badness stemmed from what my voices considered my substance or from psychiatry's ascription of it to my genes and chemistry, most things were my fault. I felt battered and assaulted by voices and welcomed damage control. Terror fueled my imprisonment, and I found my belonging and "safety" in the hospital and in psychiatrists' advice to aggressively fight the voices. I accepted huge amounts of neuroleptic drugs. Even with my treatment compliance, I acted on the commands of voices to do violence to myself and others and was repeatedly placed in seclusion where they used leather and chemical restraints and confined me in cold wet packs.

Dominant voices fought dominating professionals, and my relationship with all was subordinate and powerless. My voices were all male, as were the psychiatrists. The nurses were women, as were the aides assigned to the female ward. They carried out policy as dictated by doctors' orders for us "objects"—females and males who didn't conform to the majority view of right and wrong, health and disease. Sexuality was against policy, and physical and chemical restraints enforced principles, policy, and practice. My voices usually referred to me as "the girl," "she," "her," or "you." There was only one other female in my voice world—Hester. Hers was not a speaking voice. She was part of a legend told by voices about a key ancestor who had been burned at the stake. My fate was locked as hers had been for higher purpose—enabling the voices to reconstitute. Hector was the most dominant voice and Hester was his "twin." Voices and family/culture/religion told me that I was bad. I needed to atone, to consecrate myself through fire. They were in charge. They controlled me. My mind and body were at the disposal of nurses and aides who battled with male voices for dominion. Women patients whispered that the hospital put saltpeter in our food. Once I figured out what that meant, it seemed irrelevant. I was so filled with Thorazine, Stelazine, Haldol, Perphenazine, and other drugs, that it was hard to know if I was awake, let alone experience sexuality.

There was a rule against any physical contact. Lesbian and gay people were still diagnosed, their sexual orientation treated as an illness, but I was totally unaware. In retrospect, there were some people whom I observed sharing a connection that I now speculate was based on sexual orientation but my world then was disembodied.

After years existing in a group room with thirteen other women in a basement women's disturbed ward, I was moved with a few other women up a flight of stairs to a different ward and a smaller group room. The move unsettled me and I began seeing visions in addition to my familiar voice experiences. People's heads turned into monsters and I thought that I was back on the farm. I couldn't understand why they wouldn't allow me to do the dishes and other typical farm chores. I tried to sit in a brown chair there, attempting to find sanctuary amidst the violence and chaos. Just as my parents had tried to pry my thumb away from me, the staff considered it essential to take away my brown chair. I could hear carpenters working in the building and decided they were constructing an electric chair for my execution.

Much treatment unwittingly reenacted my hurtful experiences from childhood. Staff held me down and strapped me in restraints. I wasn't allowed to use the bathroom and had to lie in my own urine in cold wet packs. Staff were afraid of me and for me. Unexpectedly, my family took me out of the hospital against medical advice because my condition continued deteriorating and the hospital advised using ECT. My mother's cousin urged my mother to remove me and arranged for me to see a talented psychologist who met me as a human being. He later told me that he had been surprised by my resilience and strength, given my history. He held hope for me that I couldn't fathom.

That therapeutic relationship resonated with my earlier healing connections with animals and with my "adopted" farm family and with what I had dared to imagine from reading Martin Buber. That psychologist, Martin Mayman, taught me that it was safe to love and be loved regardless of outer and inner shame, fear, and violence.

As life-giving as my relationship with Dr. Mayman was, when my large doses of Thorazine and Stelazine were reduced, I started to believe he was a Nazi doctor who was having a sexual relationship with my mother. As in the hospital after the sudden ward transfer, my voice experience expanded to include horrible visions. By this time, I was working at a job I loved in the pediatrics playroom of a general hospital. It had been Dr. Mayman's hope-holding that had first allowed me to take small steps of going back to school and doing volunteer work when no other employer would hire me. I was lucky that the place that risked accepting me as a volunteer soon decided that I was worth hiring. It was work that fit me. It resonated with what I had learned to do on the farm with my "adopted" family and at their camp, my first job.

Dr. Mayman chose to ride through the storm of my terror and Nazi accusations. We continued psychotherapy without resorting to increasing my Thorazine dose. Over time, Dr. Mayman supported my learning basic trust—in myself and in him—which then generalized to others. I used my university courses to inform the work that I deeply valued. Meeting him was a lucky gift that I didn't request or earn. He was a skilled listener and a consummate teacher.

Still, my search to understand and make meaning of my experiences felt tumultuous and I sought other resources. After reading books by R. D. Laing, I wrote to him to request suggestions for "a place to be" for me. I was struggling to sustain myself at work and school while living in my parents' home and commuting for therapy with Dr. Mayman. I felt overwhelmed by emotions, lots of rage, and I sought time and space for exploration and connecting/re-connecting. Laing linked me with Loren Mosher who had started Soteria, a model research project funded by NIMH. Dr. Mosher generously sent me material to read and arranged for me to visit Soteria. Soteria was designed as a double-blind research study, and I understood that I couldn't qualify to live there as a participant; so, I was surprised when they offered me an opportunity to participate as a live-in volunteer. I felt tempted to move there but was too frightened by its apparent lack of structure. While I valued the alternative that Soteria provided and yearned to join, I had learned in therapy that external structure supported my connection to "the real" and I was too scared to try a situation apparently without structure.

As my Thorazine was reduced, I became more aware of my body and sexuality. Dr. Mayman encouraged me to think responsibly about my values and the need for birth control. He supported my growing self-respect, yet I was still repeatedly victimized. At first my encounters with men were exhilarating, though they were also unequal and hurtful. Having my feelings and body violated was familiar. I was just starting to recognize that I could set limits and say "no" when I was raped at knifepoint. Saturday night, I had gone to a movie with another student, enjoyed the evening, and rejected his invitation to spend the night. We parted on warm terms. The following afternoon I chose to go out with a man who worked at the school and whom I didn't know well. He started drinking Colt 45 and, when I rejected his advances, he got angry and pulled a knife, threatened me, and raped me. Afterward, he let me go, and I drove to Ann Arbor where Dr. Mayman worked and lived. When I phoned him, I didn't speak clearly, my distress evident. He left his son's birthday party and met me in his office. When he heard me, Dr. Mayman phoned a doctor he knew, told him that a man had "forced himself" on me, and arranged for me to receive a prescription for "the morning after pill." I didn't see the gynecologist or the police. There was no rape crisis service. I don't know whether Dr. Mayman considered that what happened to me was rape. We didn't discuss that, although I know he deeply cared about me and for me in a protective, parental way. I drove home and vomited and vomited and vomited. No one knew what had happened except the rapist, Dr. Mayman, and me. I knew that Dr. Mayman was pained that I had been hurt but I don't think he realized the limits of his understanding in this situation. I too, did not see that his lens was narrowed by his worldview as a middle-aged, white, heterosexual male psychologist and academic. My lens was also clouded, blocking my ability to see myself as an autonomous adult woman. I had accepted a less-than role as a mental patient in need of protection by others with superior knowledge, skills, and strength.

I loved my work with hospitalized children. I was in charge of the play-room on evenings and weekends. I provided a child-centered milieu—plan-ning art projects, toys, music, and stories that fit the desires and needs of the young children, and forming caring relationships with children and their families. After about two years, it seemed that a number of the children who had leukemia and other cancers were dying in greater numbers. I was strug-gling to accept my limitations and feeling increasingly unsupported by my supervisor and by the medical staff. I had dated the brother of one of the nursing assistants and he had lied to me about himself. We had been planning to get married until I broke it off. He, a black man, called me a "lily white bitch." I tried to keep the messiness of this relationship away from work but, after I ended it, I felt exposed to the judgment and gossip of the nursing staff. This coincided with my intense feelings of loss and grief at the children's deaths. My voices blamed me. I resigned. Staying at my parents' house was no longer necessary, as my purpose in living there and attending the local university was to enable me to do my work better. Without the bonds of work, I needed to move. But I was pretty stuck—unbathed, my long hair in knots, and overwhelmed.

I had written a pained letter to my old psychiatrist, the one who com-plained that it was like pulling teeth to get me to speak and had initiated my hospitalizations. Years before, he had warned against my becoming friendly with another one of his patients at the hospital by explaining that I was "good people," a bold message that his other patient was not. At seventeen years old, I had gratefully welcomed the paternal warning. This time, his response to my letter was to phone me and warn me that "the meek shall inherit the earth." He also phoned my cousin, a lawyer active in the American Civil

Liberties Union, to warn him that I should be hospitalized. Fortunately, my cousin who didn't know me well, respected my boundaries.

It was August. Dr. Mayman was away in Colorado, and I was stewing. Fortunately, my sister's best friend from college years came to visit. We knew each other, but on this visit I stayed up late talking with her husband. He and I shared our stories and formed a loving bond. The next day I finally got in the shower and accepted their help in combing out my hair tangles. They took me back to Ann Arbor where they had been staying. I slept on the floor, and the next day they went home to New Jersey. They gave me the remainder of their sublease and responsibility for cleaning and defrosting as I looked for a place to move.

I interviewed with a man who had advertised for a roommate on a nearby farm. Expectations were that we would not be sexual. There were goats to be milked and other people sharing the space and work as well. I liked them all. Despite our agreement regarding remaining nonsexual, I slept with him right away. I listened to his story and his pain. It felt more mutual than my previous relationships, but I decided that I needed more separate time and space. I didn't want a roommate. I rented a room in a man's house instead. I had house and kitchen privileges. The owner did janitorial work on the third shift at a Detroit auto factory and our paths didn't cross often.

I set about giving myself the nurturing opportunities that I had worked so hard to provide the children at the hospital. At first I had clay to sculpt. When that ran out, I borrowed books from the library and learned to bake bread. I loved flattening and kneading the dough. I walked everywhere. Dr. Mayman returned and recommended more structure, so I started swimming at the YMCA, joined a city recreation department volleyball team, and enrolled in a course titled "Children's Literature from a Developmental Perspective." It was taught by an author who was also a developmental psychologist. I continued journal and poetry writing, a practice that I had found important since adolescence. A long poem I wrote was titled, "Meaning is Movement." It was a significant and creative time for me.

As the seasons changed, I became less connected with other people and with consensual reality. I uniquely interpreted messages from the environment, including late night TV commercials. My disconnection culminated when I was in Dr. Mayman's office waiting room and he perceived me as catatonic. He tried to engage with me but I was overwhelmed by intense voices and beliefs that kept me out of his reach. My terror paralyzed me, protecting others from my violence and preventing their finding me. Dr. Mayman continued his schedule, seeing the rest of his clients. He left me on the chair and spoke to me at intervals between appointments. Finally, when he finished his work, and I was still unresponsive, Dr. Mayman phoned someone and asked him to come help. When he arrived, I heard the other man wonder why Dr. Mayman had not merely phoned for an ambulance.

They loaded me in a car and drove me to the hospital. Dr. Mayman started to explain my situation to a doctor who quickly took over and admitted me to the neuropsychiatric unit.

I was put in a bed in a room where I heard whirring. No person spoke to me. I surmised that they were filming me. I heard air circulating and believed that someone was pumping in gas to harm me. My voices warned me. I lay listening, trying to breathe in as little as possible, and unmoving for what felt like many hours. The next time I saw someone, a bevy of white coats surrounded the bed where I lay. A young man presented my body to a dominant older man. To me, the older man looked like Santa Claus except for the color of his hair and beard, which were red. Someone lifted an arm, a leg, they stayed suspended. Santa Claus explained that he would count backward from ten. I listened as he counted and then injected magic medicine. They helped move my body to a sitting positon, then to a standing position with Santa Claus supporting my left side and someone else on my right. Our odd trio began slowly walking across the room and down a hall. Santa Claus laughed and said that while most people fell asleep after receiving this medicine, it woke me up. I accepted his power. Then I returned to my earlier unmoving condition. The next time the bevy in white surrounded the bed in which my body lay, the arms and legs fell when lifted instead of remaining suspended in the air. Santa Claus asked the younger man what he had done. Self-consciously the younger man acknowledged having ordered injectable Thorazine, and Santa Claus chided him. Santa Claus periodically gave me the intravenous magic. He then instructed nurses to add a shot-glassful of liquid Haldol, which I decided was a sacrament. I concentrated on accepting the sacred communion, despite the messages from my voices.

The next turning point was when they took me to watch others play volleyball. I hadn't been talking or moving much, but once placed on the gym floor, my body reflexively moved. I joined the game and also started talking with and encouraging other players. Afterward, Neil, a psych aide, commented to me that it looked like I'd played volleyball before. That led to a conversation where I confided that I had been institutionalized and feared that I would fall back into a familiar pattern of passivity. Up to the moment when they took me off the ward to watch the game, l had surmised that I might be on a train. The hallway shape reminded me of an old train with its curved ceiling and periodic lights, including blue lights which I knew exclusively from train trips with my father. Neil advised that I explain my propensity for vegetating in hospitals the next morning at the community meeting. He explained that we were part of a therapeutic community, and I needed to request privileges and that I could explain my reasons for urging a rapid discharge. The next day, the resident psychiatrist explained that I had been committed to the hospital by a judge. He said that I would now be permitted to sign in voluntarily if I chose. I agreed to that, and then he further explained that he had another paper for me to sign. It would give them permission to use the film they had made of me for future psychiatric education. My initial distrust had correctly detected their intrusive actions, though my interpretation about their intentions had been flawed. I was inclined to sign permission, but decided to discuss it with Dr. Mayman first. He advised that I might regret doing so in the future. He still carried hope for me—hope was a strange belief he held, that I could still have a future, possibly including work, school, and love. He said that medical students who were taught by viewing my catatonia could prejudice them against seeing the fullness of me in a real-world context. I followed his advice and did not give permission for them to use the films.

After three weeks, they discharged me to a halfway house but I lasted there only a few days before my catatonic body was returned to the hospital. This time it was a young, red-headed ambulance driver who spoke toward my face lying on his gurney, "For God's sake, let them help you!" This time I was recognized by the psychiatric resident on duty in the emergency room. He was more warm and relaxed than the other doctor, but I was still returned to the same ward, staff, and "therapeutic community." It was over six months before I was again discharged, able to at least appear as if I could lead a conventional life.

My journey continued at a different college, where I finished a bachelor of philosophy degree with specializations in psychology and philosophy. I discovered feminism, enjoyed poetry, dancing, and sexual attraction to others regardless of their gender. Then I found a job in a private psychiatric hospital. I was their first woman mental health worker (and unknown to staff an ex-patient as well). The director of Nursing later explained to me that she had decided to take this risk of adding a female after years refusing to do so. It worked out, and after a couple of years there, I applied (still with psychiatric history hidden) to graduate school. I terminated therapy with Dr. Mayman for the second and final time, and traveled to Philadelphia to attend my mother's cousin's alma mater, The University of Pennsylvania School of Social Work. That summer, when I returned to visit Martin Mayman and introduced him to my future female life partner (now spouse) he responded with his usual warmth but privately doubted that I was a lesbian. In graduate school, I was active in the Feminist Social Work Collective and attempted to be an agent of change in school as well as in the wider community. I struggled and wrote to Martin Mayman, who accepted my decision to return to therapy at a feminist therapy agency. I later quit when my therapist urged me to return to psychiatric medication. I was psychiatric drug-free during 1978–1980, my two years in graduate school. That was my only time without anti-psychotic drugs until 2014 when I was able to complete weaning off of them.

I found work I loved—doing play therapy with young children. I maintained my secret identity as an ex-mental patient and was stressed by the secret-keeping. The greater my sense of being overwhelmed, the louder and harsher my voices grew. I was able to assert and advocate at work for others, especially for the less powerful, like the children and families with whom I worked, yet I lived my own life from a pretty passive position. I often resigned from jobs after psych hospital admissions, which I frequently disguised as appendectomies and other physical conditions. In 1988, I was ready to resign after a hospitalization. I had been working closely with a three-year-old boy who had been sexually abused. I experienced extreme powerlessness when a judge permitted the boy's father, whom he feared, to have unsupervised visitation with him. Nothing I did or said convinced the judge that this was not in the best interests of this child. My male psychiatrist and male agency director decided that I needed protecting and urged me to apply for short term disability rather than following my usual path of resigning. The agency's insurance policy required that I apply for Social Security Disability before they would rule on my application for short term disability. Devastated, I began my twenty-year journey identified as a person with an official disability.

My next step on the disability journey was following my psychiatrist's advice and volunteering to work with horses at a farm that offered therapeutic horseback riding. I was very clear that I wanted to do physical work caring for the horses, their barn, and pasture, and that I did not want to work with the human students there. It was a wonderful, life-giving opportunity for me. Eventually I partially forgave myself for "abandoning" my work with hurt children and healed enough to begin helping with therapeutic lessons, including those with young children. In 1993, I took the nine-month course to become certified as a therapeutic horseback riding instructor but dropped out after seven months when I was hospitalized. I had returned to full-time employment in an agency that provided mental health support. I returned to volunteering at the therapeutic riding program, and eventually applied for and completed the nine-month therapeutic instructor class and was immediately hired part-time. It was a loving environment and I thrived there; however, sometimes I left for more time in mental hospitals.

By 2006 I was assisting a friend in teaching horseback riding to participants from a mental health day program in north Philadelphia. Those students started teaching me about the Recovery Movement, prompting me to take a Recovery Foundations training. It was life changing for me. I learned that I didn't need to reach consecutive milestones before returning to more substantial work. I had been waiting for "symptom abatement," following the best advice of my mental health professionals who urged stabilizing, maintenance, and incremental steps. After the training, I suggested to the director of the Day Program that she hire me to offer story-telling workshops. She responded enthusiastically, as she was trying to re-create her program to fit Philadelphia's commitment to "Recovery Transformation." I suggested that I should take a story-telling workshop first before offering one for her program. At that training, the instructor asked me if I was interested in returning to work. I said, "yes, absolutely." She gave me the contact information for the director of an agency who was interested in hiring someone who was a person in recovery and also trained as a mental health professional. That was the beginning of a key chapter in my story and the beginning of my path to full-time meaningful work. I worked for that agency from 2007–2016. I found my voice and increasingly used it. At first, I trusted my learning and understanding about recovery, except where hearing voices was concerned. I still felt like a powerless victim in relation to my voices.

When I was asked to offer peer support with someone who was struggling with hearing voices, I knew that I was inadequate for the task. I couldn't authentically offer support to a fellow voice hearer when I felt so overwhelmed by my own voices. After struggling to eradicate fierce voices for over forty years, I discovered the Hearing Voices Network Movement and started to learn not to meet the cruel aggression of my voices with my own hostility. By assertively changing my relationship with my voices, I moved away from feeling powerless and disconnected.

Just as I learned and grew through healing connections with animals, my alternate family on the farm, nature, spirituality, and Dr. Mayman, I also needed connections with other voice-hearers to find and co-create the meaning of my voices and my life. I needed to learn to listen, to engage my voices and others with curiosity for understanding, not for cure or conquest. I had to move away from the familiar lessons, swallowed and believed for over forty years, and open to another way of listening and hearing. In the twenty-first century, the reach of my research and relationships extended quickly via the Intervoice web site and through Working to Recovery where Karen Taylor and Ron Coleman connected with me.

The Hearing Voices Network Movement taught me that the problem was not in hearing voices, but in how I reacted or responded to them. I needed enough courage to listen to their messages so that I could make sense of them and choose how to respond. First, I needed to pay attention. I set sufficient limits to enable open-hearted, open-minded hearing and also ensure physical safety for myself and others. I was accustomed to a cacophony, and I needed to sort the conglomeration into discernible notes. I began to understand that the voices were mine. They had been present for decades and their messages were particular to me and my life. I considered my life and the social, emotional, political, and cultural contexts from which my voices grew.

Feeling powerless was key in making sense of my voices. As a child, I felt terrified but unable to ask for help. An inner world formed that was populated by the Fierce. Hector was the most dominant of the Fierce. He ruled and commanded other voices and me. There were also old Gently Ones, who I thought had died out when I was seventeen. In trying to meet my voices, I asked myself whether each one was positive or negative or neutral. Initially, my answer was that they were all negative. In time, I realized that none was so absolute, that it was how I related to them that influenced whether they seemed positive or negative.

There was also a group called the Murmurers. They formed a sort of Greek chorus that raised and lowered their murmurs to fit the tone, attitudes, and commands from Hector and the other Fierce. I learned that there was nothing random about my experience. It fit my life story, and I needed to unravel the clues in order to reconstruct a more sustainable life. There was also a small group of babies who cried endlessly. I learned the names and characteristics of each discrete voice: Hector/Hester, Bert, Simon, Jasper, Billy, Benjie, Brad, and Jason.

Frankly, it was very challenging to engage with aggressive voices in an assertive yet compassionate way. It didn't feel safe or fair to relate to voices with respect when they didn't respond with equal respect. This parallels my relationships with people in my life as I have tried to learn compassionate assertiveness when passivity and/or aggression were what I had always used for survival. Like other peacemaking efforts, I needed to learn to build a peace instead of seeking to avoid mutual annihilation. One experience that enabled me to understand Hector, and therefore myself more thoroughly, was elicited by Dirk Corstens in a voice dialoguing demonstration. I had previously dialogued with all my voices by myself and had developed respectful working relationships with them but I cowered in the shadow of Hector's power and had been unable to establish a working relationship with his most dominant voice. Dirk Corstens facilitated an opening for reconstructing my understanding of honor, humility, and respect that allowed me to change my relationship with Hector and find my own center, my power from within.

The absence of war, freedom from "symptoms," does not create peace—it's freedom *for* wellness that does. When I accepted a "less-than" identity, I was willing to settle for any pacification to avoid pain and harassment. I "voluntarily" used lots of psychotropic medications and hospitalizations to avoid experiencing chaotic overwhelm. I was stuck in dualities and limiting beliefs that have dominated western medicine, economies, and society. I see our traditionally hierarchical structures as more conventionally "male," and I see more equally distributed power and shared responsibility as an approach more aligned with feminist values. I reached this vision through my process of discovering and reclaiming my power. My liberation is based on connection, interdependence, and love.

Today I am a woman firmly planted in this world—I belong! It has been an odyssey from an experience of helplessness, hopelessness, and "psychosis" to "home." My connection with other people, with myself, and with spirit grows daily as I work toward personal and societal liberation.

It is because no one heard my story for so many years that I now value telling it. I listen for and ask for other people's stories. I know the wounds caused by not being heard, seen, or understood and I also know the healing that comes from connecting with other human beings. I know the pain of caring for someone who seems barricaded and unreachable. I've stood on both sides of those silent walls and felt helpless, unable to reach and hold another person and unable to allow myself to be held. I have feared what I most desired. We know as we are known, and I learned that connecting with other people was worth the risk. I learned little by little to lower the walls to listen, hear, and speak. I did this by accepting my fear. I had to stop running long enough to get to know my fear and myself. I made fear my acquaintance, bit-by-bit, by letting myself become curious. Gradually, I was able to entertain wonder sufficiently to gain knowledge and understanding. I began to accept who I was, and that enabled me to get curious and learn about other people and the world. Curiosity is a step toward acceptance. When we accept ourselves and each other, we can choose belonging, belief, healing, and wholeness. For me, this occurred gradually. My desire to live propelled my curiosity and gave me the courage to begin connecting with other people's stories. Mutual acceptance took root. Love is an antidote to fear, and curiosity is its first expression.

Now I seek and create opportunities to practice presence—to practice being present with myself and others—to practice listening with an open heart and open mind. This is a process I started with my first breath, but my process was interrupted—interrupted by trauma and loss—by life. Such interruptions are human. They happen to everyone. The trick is to recognize them, engage with them, and make sense of them safely, so we are free to reconnect. These days, I try to create spaces that allow healing and wholeness to grow in each of us and in our communities.

REFERENCES

Eliot, T.S. (1952). "The Four Quarters: Little Gidding," in *The Complete Poems and Plays, 1909-1950*. New York: Harourt, Brace, & World.

Lorde, A. (1982). "Learning from the 60's." In *Sister Outsider: Essays and Speeches by Audre Lorde*. Berkeley: Crossing Press.

II

WOMEN, PSYCHOSIS & THE BODY

Chapter Four

Snakes in the Crib

Psychosocial Factors in Postpartum Psychosis

Marie Brown

In a series of photographs from the 1850s entitled "the physiognomy of insanity," Dr. Hugh Diamond documented the lives of patients at Surrey County Lunatic Asylum. Upon first encountering these images, I found myself struck most by one particular set. The photographs and accompanying lithograph (neatly captioned with the phrase "melancholy passing into mania") show an image of a young woman, most likely in her early-to-mid 20s, with short dark hair and a floral dress. The expression on her face is a curious one, hard to read—her eyebrows are furrowed, and with what seems almost to be a snarl, she gazes to the left looking outward over her shoulder. There is something that seems defiant about her, as if she is humoring the photographer, overturning the power of his gaze. In the accompanying text her expression is described in detail: "The eyes are not lost in vacancy; they seem to discern some person or object which excites displeasure or suspicion. The forehead is wrinkled with some strong emotion, and the eyebrows, although corrugated, have not the tense contraction toward the nose which is observable in many cases of melancholia" (Gilman, 1976, p. 48). We learn from the text that the patient came to the asylum after suffering from what was termed *puerperal mania*. The subject is described as a poor woman from London who "sorted paper" for a meager living. Her symptoms lasted for six months subsequent to giving birth, and during this time she spoke incoherently and declared that her infant did not belong to her. After this period of initial confused excitation, she became despondent—not moving for long periods of time, unable to speak. After another six months, she fell back into wild mania, began to dress herself "fantastically," sang songs, and developed a preoccupation with ideas of "wealth and pleasure" (p. 45).

Strange to say, but what is perhaps most remarkable about these images is simply that they acknowledge postpartum psychosis as worthy of documentation. Here, it is seen as an infliction in its own right, a category that is given name and labeled in ink, something to be documented, learned about, and understood. This is striking given that postpartum psychosis has made only fleeting appearances across the history of psychology and psychiatry. It is scarcely mentioned in textbooks on reproductive psychiatric disorders or even by more contemporary feminist theorists. There is hardly a glimpse of it in psychoanalysis and almost none in sociology. For example, Jane Ussher's seminal text *Managing the Monstrous Feminine*, despite its rich and critical analysis of the psychiatric reproductive body, gives scant mention of postpartum psychosis other than to link it to a biological disposition[1] Likewise, contemporary researchers making advances in the psychosocial understanding of psychosis often neglect to include psychosis in the postpartum. In Simon McCarthy-Jones's well-researched and cutting-edge book *Hearing Voices: The Histories, Causes, and Meanings of Auditory Verbal Hallucinations,* voice-hearing is described at length in people diagnosed with schizophrenia spectrum disorders, bipolar disorder, major depressive disorder, post-traumatic stress disorder, dissociative identity disorder, borderline personality disorder, epilepsy, addiction, Parkinson's disease, Alzheimer's disease, brain traumas, deafness, and healthy populations as well as analyzed historically, phenomenologically, spiritually, cross-culturally, and neurologically. However, despite its impressive breadth of inquiry, postpartum hallucinations are only referenced in passing and merely to assert the disorder's rarity.[2] This begs the question of what might be behind this silence as well as what may be motivating and maintaining it. Is postpartum psychosis really so rare that it fails to justify more substantial engagement? I would like to suggest that the cause of this silence reflects the fashion in which postpartum psychosis involves two identities most overlooked by Western society: those whom we call "psychotic" and those whom we call mothers.

Although many disciplines, particularly clinical psychology, are interested in the effect of mothers on their children's well-being, there is a curious lack of interest in mothers themselves. Rarely are mothers seen as subjects in their own right. The "Where Are Mothers?" Project (WAM), conducted by researchers at the Maternal Psychology Laboratory at Teachers College Columbia University, was a large-scale, systematic review of the current state of scholarly literature on mothers in the areas of women and psychology, developmental psychology, clinical psychology, social psychology, psychiatry, nursing, and obstetrics/gynecology. Strikingly, across these disciplines, out of 75,282 original research articles published in forty-seven journals in the past two decades, only 5.6 percent studied mothers as a population of interest. One of the most influential publications in the field of clinical psychology, the *Journal of Clinical Psychology*, devoted only 0.8 percent of its articles to the subject of motherhood. Even in the subfield of women and psychology, an inherently female-focused discipline, only about 5 percent of the total number of articles published were on mothers. In *Psychology of Women Quarterly*, a leading journal in women's psychology, only 3.6 percent of its publications where on mothers. The WAM authors conclude, "Even though mothers can be traced back to the roots of all social, psychological, and physiological theories on human development, they have not been recognized as subjects of interest to study in their own right, with many leading and respected journals devoting less than 1 percent of all articles to the investigation of their wellbeing" (Athan et al., 2013). It is important to view these findings with an understanding of just how many women are mothers—in the United States alone, 43.5 million women are mothers (U.S. Census Bureau, 2012). In sum, there is a serious lack of literature on motherhood, and particularly with respect to the mothers' subjective experiences.

Likewise, the most prominent voices in scholarship concerning psychosis often focus less on the subjective experiences of individuals, and more on neuroscientific, genetic, or biological concerns. Although there has been some paradigmatic shift, the majority of fully-funded and institutionally-sanctioned research on psychosis still relies on nomothetic approaches, symptom checklists, and raw biological data.[3] Popular perceptions of psychosis and schizophrenia increasingly assume the etiological primacy of biology (Pescosolido et al., 2010). Although there is merit in biomedical approaches, the overwhelming domination of their voices in discourse essentially silences the subjects of their inquiry, leading to the systematic erasure of the actual experience of psychosis as it has been lived by individuals. Therefore, much like with mothers, people with psychosis are often only indirectly subjects of scientific and theoretical inquiry, their own subjective experiences neglected.

With the relative lack of academic concern for the subjective experience both of mothers and people experiencing psychosis, the scarcity of scholarship on postpartum psychosis is hardly surprising. Feminist scholars seeking to deconstruct purely biomedical approaches to reproductive and maternal mental health (e.g., premenstrual syndrome, postpartum depression), may not have knowledge regarding critical, survivor, or service-user approaches to psychosis. Likewise, psychosis researchers with a psychosocial emphasis may have limited knowledge of feminist scholarship, and may not recognize mothers as important subjects of inquiry. Thus, the understanding of postpartum psychosis from a critical and psychosocial perspective can be expected to offer something both for scholars of feminism and psychosis.

The contemporary research on the etiology of postpartum psychosis that does exist primarily relies on the biomedical model. Specifically, the occurrence of postpartum psychosis is commonly attributed to hormonal shifts after birthing. The popularity of these hormonal theories, coupled with the

general absence of psychological explanations, reflects wider social discourses that pathologize the female reproductive body. For example, hormonal theories of postpartum psychosis strongly parallel popular conceptions of
the "unruly hormones" of premenstrual syndrome. These theories cast the
female reproductive body as unstable, chaotic, and irrational, particularly in
contrast to male bodies. In speaking of the reproductive psychiatric disorders
of premenstrual syndrome and postnatal depression, Ussher (2006) states,
"the problem is located within: the monster in the machine of femininity
positioned as endocrine or neurotransmitter dysfunction, or 'female sex hormones,' a pathology within the woman, outside of her control (but within the
control of medical experts, we are assured)" (p. 17). Therefore, women who
experience postpartum psychosis can be understood as subject to two areas of
thought that delegitimize their own power and control—firstly through viewing the female body as fundamentally dysfunctional, and secondly by regarding psychosis as solely the product of faulty brain or body chemistry. It might
be noted that self-agency, or a sense of "control," has been posited as an
important component of recovery from schizophrenia and other psychotic
disorders (Farkas, 2007; Lieberman et al., 2008; Rashed, 2015); as well as a
predictor of greater quality of life in people experiencing psychotic symptoms, such as auditory hallucinations (Hansen, Vakhrusheva, Khan, Ramirez.
& Kimhy, 2016). For this reason, the way in which the dominant discourse
understands postpartum psychosis is gravely important for women suffering
from the experience.

Relying solely on biomedical discourse fails to allow room for functional
explanations of postpartum psychosis and forestalls the development of
psychosocial treatments and approaches. To date, there are no psychotherapeutic techniques or methods specifically geared toward women experiencing psychosis in the postpartum. This is despite the existence of a new mother's complex needs, such as the continued ability to care-take and breastfeed
their children. In addition, as postpartum psychosis is a gender-specific disorder, the fashion in which we understand this phenomenon has direct implications for how we view women more generally. With respect to medical
representations of women's "faulty hormones" and "reproductive distress,"
Ussher (2006) states, "This has significant implications for the ways in which
we, as women, inhabit our bodies, for knowledge about what our bodies are,
and what they are meant to do, materializes in our experience of our fecund
flesh, more broadly, in the development of our subjectivity, our sense of
ourselves as women" (p. 17). Therefore, the manner in which we understand
postpartum psychosis is intimately linked to the ways in which women view
themselves and their bodies more broadly. Hormonal representations of postpartum psychosis cast the reproductive body as disconnected from the self—
as an entity to be feared and controlled by outside professionals.

Similarly, the overreliance on hormonal theories of postpartum psychosis does a disservice to progressive and alternative theories on psychosis more generally. If postpartum psychosis can occur within a biomedical vacuum of hormonal dysregulation, so too can psychoses more generally. This is problematic in that it neglects the role of psychosocial factors in the development of psychosis, such as living in a densely populated urban area (Vassos, Pedersen, Murray, Collier, & Lewis, 2012), poverty (Werner, Malaspina, & Rabinowitz, 2007), race (Schwartz & Blankenship, 2014), and immigration (Weiser et al., 2008). Importantly, theories on psychosis, biological or otherwise, should be informed by an intersectional perspective, recognizing that social identities such as gender, race, and class, and their concomitant systems of oppression are impossible to disentangle from issues of mental health, as each individual is subject to multiple and overlapping politics of identity. Taking a more philosophical perspective on the body, Grosz (1994) states:

> I am not suggesting that medical, biological, even chemical analyses of bodies are "wrong" or "inappropriate"; my claim is the simpler one that the guiding assumptions and prevailing methods used by these disciplines (indeed, by any discipline), have tangible effects on the bodies studied. Bodies are not inert; they function interactively and productively. They act and react. They generate what is new, surprising, unpredictable. (p. *xi*)

Likewise, this chapter takes a dynamic and interactional perspective towards postpartum psychosis, stressing that the ways in which we speak about and understand "the psychotic" or "the female" body affects bodies themselves, both as within their physicality and in the ways in which they are experienced by the people who inhabit them. To this end, this chapter seeks to understand the current knowledge on postpartum psychosis and the ways in which scholarship can be expanded to present a more holistic understanding of experience. While this chapter is not meant to be an exhaustive report on postpartum psychosis, key findings and theories will be described across epidemiology and risk factors, diagnostic questions, symptom presentation, historical perspectives, treatment, and recovery, as well as discussions on the role of self-disturbance, infanticide, and spirituality. My purpose is to bring the subject of postpartum psychosis into conversation with both feminist scholarship and progressive psychosis research.

EPIDEMIOLOGY AND RISK FACTORS

Postpartum psychosis affects 1 to 2 of every 1,000 deliveries (Kendell, Chalmers, & Platz, 1987; Munk-Olsen, Laursen, Pedersen, Mors, & Mortensen, 2006). For sake of comparison, this is the same rate of occurrence as

Down Syndrome (Twomey, 2012), a fact that problematizes the frequent reports of the "rarity" of the disorder. In fact, in the two years following pregnancy, women have a four-fold increase in the likelihood of being hospitalized due to a psychotic disorder (Bokhari, Bhatara, Bandettini, & McMillin, 1998). More generally, women are more likely to be admitted to a psychiatric unit after giving birth than at any other time in their lives (Doucet, Dennis, Letourneau, & Blackmore, 2009).

There are several risk factors associated with postpartum psychosis. Some evidence suggests it is most common in women with a prior diagnosis of bipolar disorder, with many researchers believing postpartum psychosis to be integrally linked to bipolarity (Jones & Craddock, 2001). However, in a cohort study of women presenting with postpartum psychosis, only 33 percent of women had an antecedent history of bipolar disorder (Blackmore et al., 2013), suggesting the connection between bipolarity and postpartum psychosis may be overstated. The likelihood of postpartum psychosis has also been found to be much higher in those with other psychotic diagnoses such as schizophrenia (Kendell et al., 1987) and schizoaffective disorders[4] (Jones & Craddock, 2001). Primipara, or first-time, mothers have a greater risk of experiencing postpartum psychosis (Kisa, Aydemir, Kurt, Gulen, & Goka, 2007), as well as older mothers (ages 40–44) (Nager, Johansson, & Sundquist, 2005). However, more recent studies have actually come to the opposite conclusion, with youth (18–25 years) more associated with postpartum psychosis than relative maturity (Upadhyaya, Sharma, & Raval, 2014).

Socioeconomic status (SES) has robustly been associated with postpartum psychosis across epidemiological research. Women with low SES or who are living in impoverished communities have an increased likelihood of postpartum psychosis (Nager, Johansson, & Sundquist, 2006). This finding is consistent with other forms of psychosis, including schizophrenia and schizoaffective disorder. Interestingly, experiences during pregnancy and delivery have also been associated with postpartum psychosis, including difficult delivery, Caesarean section, and shorter gestation period (Kendell et al., 1987). Sharma, Smith, and Khan (2004) found that women with postpartum psychosis had longer labors and were more likely to have delivered at night. Blackmore et al., (2006) found that experiencing a complication during delivery more than doubled a mother's risk for postpartum psychosis. In addition, having a female baby (Agrawal, Bhatia, & Malik, 1990) and stressful life events (Lopez et al., 2008) have all been associated with increased risk. Upadhyaya et al. (2014) found that the five main risks for developing postpartum psychosis are youth, lower per capita income, perinatal complications, neonatal complications, and the absence of a partner during the peripartum phase. All of these risk factors may set an individual up for less resilience in the face of trauma or significant stressors (such as birthing). Given this, what is most striking about the literature on risk factors is the absence of trauma as a clearly-defined variable of interest in postpartum psychosis. This is particularly important given the high association between traumatic life events and various psychosis outcomes, including increased risk of psychotic disorders and prodromal psychosis, as well as attenuated positive psychotic symptoms (Gibson, Alloy, & Ellman, 2016). This is especially important to consider given that complicated, difficult births and pregnancies, as well as neonatal complications, are risk factors for postpartum psychosis. Although the literature discusses these factors as predictors of postpartum psychosis, these experiences are often understood in terms of biological or physiological impact (such as insomnia) rather than their psychological impact. Therefore, more information is needed regarding the potential relationship between postpartum psychosis and traumatic birth and pregnancy experiences from a psychological perspective.

DIAGNOSIS

The diagnosis of postpartum psychosis has historically been fraught with debate. Across time, it has been known by several names, including puerperal psychosis, puerperal insanity, lactation insanity, postpartum bipolar disorder, and puerperal mania, among others. There has been a longstanding dispute in the psychiatric field concerning whether postpartum psychosis should be considered as a distinct diagnosis in and of itself, or the occurrence of an already underlying mental disorder triggered by childbirth. The current issues of both the *Diagnostic and Statistical Manual of Mental Disorders* (*DSM-5*) and *International Classification of Diseases* (*ICD-10*), do not provide diagnostic criteria specifically for postpartum psychosis. Therefore, mothers experiencing symptoms of psychosis are first diagnosed with another disorder, and then given a specifier to indicate a connection between childbirth and the onset of symptoms. It was not until the release of *DSM-IV* in 1994 that an onset specifier was included as a means to demarcate the postpartum period as meaningful. The specifier for *DSM-IV* was: "with postpartum onset: defined as within four weeks of delivering a child" (American Psychiatric Association [APA], 2000). This specifier could be added to an overarching diagnosis of Major Depressive Disorder, Manic or Mixed Episode of Major Depressive Disorder, Bipolar Mood Disorder, or Brief Psychotic Disorder. For example, a mother experiencing psychotic symptoms after childbirth can be diagnosed with "Brief Psychotic Disorder with peripartum onset"—meaning that she must meet the criteria for Brief Psychotic Disorder in order to be considered as having the colloquial "postpartum psychosis" or she can be given a diagnosis of Major Depressive Disorder with psychotic features, Bipolar I, Schizoaffective, or Unspecified Functional Psychosis (Doucet et al., 2009). With the release of the *DSM-5*, the onset specifier was changed to "with peripartum onset" (APA, 2013). This change in terminology is significant in that it now includes the period of time during pregnancy as well as the postpartum period. However, this specifier still only indicates the short time window of four weeks after delivery (APA, 2013). If symptoms occur during pregnancy or in the four weeks after delivery, the specifier can be added to a Major Depressive Disorder, Bipolar I or Bipolar II. In sum, the *DSM-5* currently assumes postpartum psychosis to be a mood or psychotic disorder triggered by pregnancy or childbirth.

The *International Classification of Diseases* has had a similarly confusing history regarding diagnostic criteria for postpartum psychosis. It appeared as a diagnosis in the 1979 edition (*ICD-8*) only to disappear in subsequent editions. The replacement category has been described by Jones and Smith (2009) as "only a ragbag [of] mental and behavioural disorders associated with the puerperium, not elsewhere classified available for episodes with onset within 6 weeks of delivery and only if they do not meet the criteria for disorders classified elsewhere" (p. 412). Therefore, although the term "postpartum psychosis" is used colloquially, there is no formal diagnosis. Importantly, others who experience psychotic symptoms after the four-to-six-week time frame of the specifier will be diagnosed without any indication of childbirth onset. This is problematic for at least two main reasons: 1) diagnosing women without a peripartum specifier limits the ability of researchers and clinicians to understand and explore the role childbirth or pregnancy may have played in the development of symptoms, and 2) women will be diagnosed with longer-term conditions, such as schizophrenia or bipolar disorder, leading to innumerable negative sequela associated with diagnosis more broadly. For example, for a woman given a longer-term diagnosis, her chances of being prescribed long-term antipsychotics may greatly increase and she may experience a sense of hopelessness and chronicity, leading to the development of an identity as a "patient" or a person who is "mentally ill." Not acknowledging the role of childbirth, and instead labeling mothers with a longer-term or "severe" mental disorder, may also impact other people's perceptions of her capacity to mother. This may in turn lead to familial, social, or legal difficulties. She may also go on to develop her own internalized stigma, causing her to doubt her own capabilities to mother or otherwise function productively. This is particularly problematic in that mothers often first experience symptoms beyond the first four-to-six weeks, with many researchers suggesting the time period should be extended two-to-six months postpartum (Sharma & Mazmanian, 2014). Postpartum psychosis as an experience without a diagnosis exists at a complicated intersection. On the one hand, a discrete diagnosis may provide greater clarification and understanding of the experience of postpartum psychosis by highlighting its connection to birth/pregnancy yet, on the other hand, insisting on a diagnosis may lead to the reification of it as a biological "illness" without psychosocial factors.

SYMPTOMS

More information is needed about the phenomenology of postpartum psychosis and the ways in which it does and does not differ from other forms of psychosis. To date, there have been few systematic comparisons between psychotic symptoms in other disorders, and psychotic symptoms in postpartum psychosis. In fact, most studies of the phenomenology of postpartum psychosis occurred during the nineteenth century, with few having been carried out in recent times—particularly when compared to the amount of attention paid by researchers to other psychotic disorders such as schizophrenia, bipolar disorder or schizoaffective disorder.

Many researchers describe symptom onset as sudden and unexpected, occurring forty-eight hours to two weeks after giving birth. However, other researchers have reported a symptom-free period during the first forty-eight hours postpartum (Doucet et al., 2009). Consistent with current specifiers, the majority of cases are thought to occur within the first two-to-four weeks after childbirth (Ebeid, Nassif, & Sinha, 2010), however this is not always the case. Mood lability is thought to progress into psychotic symptoms including, delusions, hallucinations, and disorganization. Some researchers consider the core feature of postpartum psychosis to be mania, with many mothers fluctuating between elation and rapid depression (Doucet et al., 2009). Symptoms can also include restlessness, agitation, sleep disturbance, paranoia, disorganized thinking, catatonia, and impulsivity (Focht & Kellner, 2012).

Similarly, Klompenhouwer et al. (1995) methodically analyzed the day to day descriptions of the behavior and utterances of 281 women admitted to the mother and baby unit at the Rotterdam University Hospital. They gathered information from detailed nurse's reports, which included symptom presentation, content of conversations, and the mothers' attitudes toward their babies and others. These researchers found that women experiencing postpartum psychosis experienced symptoms phenomenologically distinct from schizophrenia and other psychoses. For example, they found that 88 percent of the women studied had experienced a "disturbance of consciousness" in the days and weeks leading up to their psychotic break. This disturbance of consciousness is characterized by fluctuating periods of disorientation and confusion, with most mothers having full or partial amnesia when retrospectively asked about this time period. The researchers conclude that this is distinctly different than the clinical picture of schizophrenia and more on course with an affective psychosis.

HISTORICAL PERSPECTIVES

Tovino (2010), in a comprehensive review of postpartum illness from antiquity to the present day, attributes the earliest depictions of postpartum psychosis to Hippocrates, who, in 400 B.C. described a case of postpartum insomnia, which progressed into psychosis. Tovino states that the first comprehensive studies of postpartum illness did not occur until the nineteenth century, at which time illnesses were classified according to their relationship to pregnancy (i.e., gestation), puerperal (within six weeks of childbirth), or lactational (occurring after six weeks). Early theories from the Salpêtrière attributed "postpartum insanity" to women's failure (or rejection) of nursing, known as the "suppression-of-milk" theory. In the second half of the nineteenth century, British physician George Fielding Blandford, attributed postpartum psychosis to the opposite—*excessive* nursing.

In England during the Victorian era, 7 to 10 percent of female asylum admissions were said to be the result of "puerperal insanity" (Showalter, 1985). Showalter (1985) describes the way in which these women violated Victorian conceptions of maternity and femininity. Specifically, these women were "indifferent to the usual conventions of politeness and decorum in speech, dress, and behavior; their deviance covered a wide spectrum from eccentricity to infanticide" (p. 58). During the Victorian era, women, and especially mothers, were expected to be modest; in contrast, puerperal insanity was associated with obscenity, sexuality, and masturbation. In fact, many physicians questioned if puerperal insanity was actually a return to the "natural state" of women previously kept under wraps by social, religious, and moral control (Showalter, 1987). In this way, postpartum insanity was seen as opening a Pandora's box of women's depravity, a box needed to be kept closed through social order.

Although not tied directly to birthing, during the 1900s, Eugen Bleuler spoke of the existence of "governess psychoses" (Noll, 2000, p. 150). This form of psychosis was seen as an occupational hazard—a form of *dementia praecox* derived from being a governess to children of wealthy parents. The existence of this form of psychosis is interesting in that a governess is an "allomother" therefore, removing the birthing experience (and therefore hormonal component) of postpartum psychosis. Bleuler believed that the disease of governess psychosis arose from a combination between inhumane treatment by employers and a desire in these young women to rise above their social standing while lacking the means to do so. This line of thinking could easily be expanded to include all personal desires to do something other than care-take children while existing within a patriarchal society that demands a commitment on women to mother.

In Karl Jaspers's landmark publication, *General Psychopathology*, psychosis produced by childbirth is given a small entry under the more

general section of "sexual epochs and reproduction." He states, "The reproductive processes (pregnancy, the puerperium, and lactation) bring psychic
disturbances along with the total change in the organism. In so-disposed
women they are sometimes the cause or the precipitating factor for psychosis
proper" (Jaspers, 1923/1963, p. 629). He goes on to cite Kraepelin, who
believed that over 14 percent of all mental disturbances in women are
"psychoses of reproduction." Jaspers believed that postpartum psychosis was
caused by constitutional and genetic factors, rather than as a direct result of
pregnancy itself. His rationale was that the psychic shifts that the majority of
pregnant women experience (e.g., mood lability, hypersensitivity to the environment, etc.) are completely uninfluential in the exacerbation of psychosis
in women with postpartum psychosis. As mentioned previously, this thinking
regarding postpartum psychosis is in keeping with current biomedical discourses, which see postpartum psychosis as indicative of an already underlying mood disorder.

Based in the UK, Action on Postpartum Psychosis (PP) is the leading
advocacy group for postpartum psychosis. This organization is innovative, in
that their Experts by Experience program offers peer specialist support to
women experiencing postpartum psychosis, as well as a collection of first-
person accounts on their webpage. However, Action on PP only stresses
biological factors of postpartum psychosis. In a pamphlet written for women
at high risk for postpartum psychosis they state,

> There are likely to be many factors that lead to an episode of PP [postpartum
> psychosis]. Research points to genetic factors and biological changes around
> the time of pregnancy and childbirth. You are more likely to have PP if a close
> relative has had it, or if you have Bipolar Disorder or Schizoaffective Disor-
> der. Changes in hormone levels and disrupted sleep patterns after giving birth
> may also be involved, but more research is needed to fully understand the
> causes. PP is not your or your partner's fault. It is not caused by anything you
> or your partner have thought or done. Relationship problems, or the baby
> being unwanted do not cause PP. (Action on Postpartum Psychosis, 2014, p. 4)

However, as previously mentioned in this chapter, empirical research tells
a different story, as psychosocial risk factors, including relationship problems, lack of social support, and poverty have all been associated with postpartum psychosis. Although an important advocacy organization, their mate-
rials can be critiqued for their limited acknowledgment of psychosocial risk
factors, including complicated birth, poverty, and immigration, among others. Currently, no advocacy organization seeks to promote a more holistic
perspective of postpartum psychosis.

FIRST-PERSON ACCOUNTS

The only way we can understand more about the experience of postpartum psychosis is by listening to the accounts of those who have lived through it. Perhaps the most famous first-person account of postpartum psychosis is Charlotte Perkins Gilman's *The Yellow Wallpaper*, a work that has become part of the canon of Women's and Gender Studies literature. Although considered a work of fiction, *The Yellow Wallpaper* was based on Gilman's own mental health experiences. Arguably, the work can be considered almost a precursor to the psychiatric survivor movement. Gilman states that her text was written in order to teach her physician, Dr. S. Weir Mitchell, "the error of his ways" (quoted in Thrailkill, 2002, p. 528). Similarly, Gilman has said the text was "not intended to drive people crazy, but to save people from being crazy" (quoted in Thrailkill, 2002, p. 527). Therefore, Gilman's writing is much more than an entertaining Gothic tale of madness, but a purposeful text that critiques medical approaches to women's mental health and comments on the patriarchal oppression of women, particularly as a result of their reproductive bodies and socially enforced caretaking social roles.

Gilman's story is a fascinating insight into the experience of one individual's subtle emersion into psychosis; the text making gentle shifts toward a confusion between self and other, between "sanity" and "insanity." In the story, the narrator is a recent mother who is experiencing psychological distress described generically as a "nervous condition." It is clear that the onset of her difficulties seems to have coincided with the birth of her child, who is a young infant at the time of the story. The narrator is confined to an old nursey inside of a colonial vacation home by her husband, John, a physician. Although a creative woman, she is prohibited from writing due to her psychological condition. She tells us about her days in short fragments that we understand to have been written quickly before anyone notices. The narrator becomes increasingly fascinated by the yellow wallpaper in the nursery. She spends her days absorbed in the pattern, color, texture, and smell of the wallpaper. As she looks at the wallpaper, she begins to see the image of a woman trapped behind the paper. In Gilman's *The Yellow Wallpaper* the narrator's so-called symptoms are understood as meaningful representations of her current struggles. Much like the Hearing Voices approach, which seeks to understand the message behind what is commonly termed "psychosis," the content of the visions of the protagonist in *The Yellow Wallpaper* give insight into the problems that lie beneath her experience. Similar to the woman she sees trapped behind the nursery wallpaper, the protagonist is trapped, both in her role as mother and, quite literally, in the nursery where she has been confined by her husband.

Contemporarily, there are a vast number of first-person accounts of postpartum psychosis available as self-published works or from small publishers, including titles such as: *A Mother's Climb Out of Darkness* by Jennifer Hentz Moyer; *From Shattered Dreams: My Journey Through Postpartum Psychosis* by Dorothy R. Ruhwald; and *Insanity's Shoes: My Running Trip Through Postpartum Psychosis* by Angela Tompkins. What all these books have in common is a yearning to share knowledge about postpartum psychosis and a desire to shed light on an experience that was not understood, both by the authors themselves as they were experiencing it, and by the healthcare providers they came in contact with.

Similar to the sentiments of many first-person accounts of madness, many of these narratives critique the treatment received while in care, particularly during crises. For example, Moyer, the author of *A Mother's Climb Out of Darkness* states:

> Looking back now, I can see how much of my fear might have been alleviated if the people who treated me had explained what was happening. Even today, I'm not sure why they didn't. Perhaps they thought I was unable to understand. But I can tell you for sure that explanations would have helped. Being treated with dignity and respect would have helped. Medication alone was not enough. (p. 25)

Beth: A Story of Postpartum Psychosis by Shirley Cervene Halvorson is a first-person account by a mother whose daughter develops psychosis in the postpartum and suicides. Keeping in mind the psychosocial risk factors previously noted by the empirical literature, we can more clearly see the same themes emerging in the text. For example, Beth is described as having a difficult birthing experience, both due to physical demands of the act, as well as the neglectful and callous treatment by her physicians. However, unlike the predominant discourse regarding risk factors, Beth's mother directly describes the experience as *psychologically* traumatic. She states,

> The doctor remained in the hall where I sought him out about two hours later. I asked him how long he was going to leave her like this. "Oh, about 3 hours," he said. It was now 3:00 am. Hard labor had begun about 9:00pm- six hours earlier. She had been in bed since the morning. His lack of caring must have been traumatic to Beth. (p. 13)

The doctor eventually needs to use instruments in order to deliver the baby, resulting in excessive vaginal bleeding of which Beth is not notified. Her mother states:

> On the fifth day, she discovered she was packed full of gauze from excessive bleeding during the birth . . . The doctor had not even told her about the gaze, and she discovered it and removed it. She said, "I am so mad at my doctor for not even telling me about the gaze, I am done with him . . . " (p. 19)

The book continues to described similar treatment once Beth is hospitalized for psychotic symptoms. Her mother describes the mental health staff as
unknowledgeable, disinterested, and condescending toward her daughter.
Beth is given electroconvulsive therapy, which temporarily seems to improve
her condition, but is abruptly discontinued after it leads her to "speak in
tongues." Beth is also forced by staff to learn "mothering skills" (p. 45). She
is placed alone in a room with her baby, Kyle, and given a bottle, diapers,
formula, and a playpen. Her mother states:

> She had not taken care of this baby for three months. How was she supposed to
> do it now? This was not an educational experience! Beth was totally petrified
> when this happened. . . . This appeared to be very traumatic for her, because
> when I arrived home, she was on the phone with [her husband] begging him to
> come for Kyle. *She had been set up for failure.* (p. 45–46; italics in original)

Although the book depicts events that took place during the late 1980s, there
are still no formal guidelines for postpartum psychosis treatment.

INFANTICIDE

Public discourse on postpartum psychosis, much like with other forms of
"mental illness," often revolves around issues of violence, specifically, infanticide. In fact, postpartum psychosis is rarely acknowledged publically until
sparked by media coverage of a women who has murdered or attempted to
harm her child. One recent example is the case of thirty-four-year-old Miriam Carey, which sparked massive media coverage in the United States after
she drove her car through a security barrier at the White House, prompting a
high-speed chase, eventually resulting in her death by police fire. In the car
with her was her eighteen-month old infant daughter. Carey was reported to
have been experiencing depression after the birth of her daughter as well as
beliefs regarding President Obama and electronic monitoring of her home
(Rendon, 2013). The story prompted interest by the American Psychological
Association (APA), who responded to the media maelstrom with a blog post
titled "There Are No Words: Postpartum Mood Disorders and Miriam Carey's Death." The author of the piece, psychologist Walker Karraa, used the
occasion to illuminate the neglect of the mental health field to develop a
language with which to discuss postpartum mood disorders. She stated,

> And as the news media looked to professionals for insight, there was mass
> confusion as to what to actually call "it." Psychosis? Depression? The only
> common denominator was the word, "postpartum" [. . .] While mood disor-
> ders around childbearing have been recorded since Hippocrates, providers and
> society have yet to agree upon a word, or collection of words that defines
> diagnoses, much less a differential one. (Karraa, 2013)

However, this was not the first time that such a response occurred. In June 2001, Andrea Yates, a Texas woman, drowned her five children during an episode of postpartum psychosis in which she believed she was possessed by Satan. Afterward, a piece written by *Seattle Times* columnist Lynne Varner (2002) stated:

> I hadn't planned to write about Andrea Yates again. But then I found out that postpartum psychosis occurs in 1 out of 1,000 births. If it were any other disease, we'd be doing 5K runs to raise awareness. I hate thinking about what Andrea Yates did, much less the reasons why. But 1 out of 1,000 women and their families deserve help, not silence.

That the silence surrounding postpartum psychosis is only occasionally broken by instances of infanticide is perhaps indicative of a society in which the needs of infants are given precedence over mothers themselves. In Hyman's (2004) article on Andrea Yates, she states:

> Cases of maternal infanticide are gripping because they seem to violate an inherent natural law, calling into question the essentialist notion that women are endowed with a nurturing maternal instinct. Incidences of maternal infanticide garner more press than paternal infanticide and evoke greater outrage from the public. (p. 192)

She goes on to compare the news coverage of Yates's case with that of Adair Garcia, a man who similarly killed five of his children. More than 1,150 articles were written about Yates, yet only 77 on Garcia. Postpartum psychosis can be understood as bearing the weight of both the public's fascinated-repulsion with maternal killing and already existing popularized connections between psychosis and violence. This combination affects not only media representations of postpartum psychosis, but also public advocacy.

The focus on a connection between infanticide and postpartum psychosis also occurred during the Victorian era. Interestingly, during this time period infanticide was not seen as merely the end result of a biologically-driven "madness," but as having psychosocial triggers as well. Showalter (1987) notes that at the time, judges and juries presiding over cases understood infanticide as connected to poverty, domestic violence, and "illegitimate" children—rarely occurring in middle-class households. However, more contemporary writings on postpartum psychosis seem to disregard this connection, instead viewing infanticide as a danger caused exclusively by "the illness." For example, in the only theoretical book solely dedicated to the subject of postpartum psychosis, *Understanding Postpartum Psychosis: A Temporary Madness,* author Teresa M. Twomey continually draws the connection between postpartum psychosis and infanticide. In her introduction, she states the reason she wrote the book was "*Saving the lives of babies and mothers*" (p. *xv*), a statement which directly connects postpartum psychosis to loss of life. She later states, "In some ways it is surprising that over 90 percent of these women *do not* harm anyone. Yet, we continue to act shocked when tragedy occurs when these ill women are left to care for babies" (p. *xx*). Statements such as these contain a curious "doublespeak" regarding the potential for violence in women with postpartum psychosis, it is at once described as rare, yet still considered unsurprising. Unfortunately, discourse such as this perpetuates negative stereotypes connecting psychosis and violence and provides an unnuanced perspective of infanticide. That is, infanticide is seen as a blanket threat for all women with postpartum psychosis, irrespective of sociocultural factors. One reason for this may be the complicated question of guilt. Twomey (2009) directly acknowledges this in her book as she quotes the following statement, "It makes no sense to hold someone responsible for a neurochemical event that is out of her control" (p. 34). Statements such as these beg the question, can we really "blame" mothers for difficult circumstances either? Why the reliance on biology to supersede blame? In *Infanticide: Psychosocial and Legal Perspectives on Mothers Who Kill*, the women responsible for infant homicides include mothers younger than seventeen years of age with more than one child, no prenatal care, and low maternal education level (i.e., not completing high school). Postpartum psychosis was not listed as a major contributor to infanticide over and above these factors. Therefore, the connection between infanticide and postpartum psychosis should be significantly reduced (however not neglected), as well as explained with a more nuanced understanding, including social context. Conflating postpartum psychosis with infanticide/violence is problematic, however the failure to recognize the risk entirely is also problematic; a balance needs to be met in future discourse.

SELF-DISTURBANCE

Self-disturbance is a theme with potentially significant implications for the understanding of postpartum psychosis. Although not formally listed as criterion in the *DSM-5*, self-disturbance has long been recognized as a central feature of psychosis (Nelson & Raballo, 2015). Self-disturbance was originally referred to as an inability to maintain "ego boundaries" (Benedetti, 1987, p. 3) by Freud's contemporary, Paul Federn. The term later came to be inclusive of all phenomenon in which there is a blurring of the boundary between the self and the outside world. In people diagnosed with schizophrenia, self-disturbance is seen as manifesting itself in a number of ways, including a weakened ability to maintain a first-person perspective or sense of "I," depersonalization, identity confusion, and disturbed self/other boundaries (Nelson, Parnas, & Sass, 2014).

McWilliams (2015) describes the "hallmark" of psychotic experience as "an inability to discriminate inside from outside" and recognizes "merger with others dominates experience, and because of an ongoing sense of separate selfhood has not been fully achieved, annihilation anxiety is pervasive" (p. 66). This is in keeping with the developmental tier model of Kernberg, who views the primary developmental task of infancy as a psychical demarcation between self and other, with the failure to do so conceived as the developmental precursor to the emergence of psychotic symptomatology.

Definitions of pathology and mental health often rely on a continuum of self-other distinction. Psychosis is thus considered as the most extreme form of pathology, this being determined by a poorly-developed self-concept and a lack of strong boundaries between self and other, inside and outside. This view of psychopathology also tends to cast psychosis as the consequence of a "developmental arrest." The concept of self-disturbance in psychosis is particularly relevant to postpartum manifestations because, based on the sheer physicality of the experience, motherhood, birthing, and pregnancy are rife with instances of self-disturbance. In my prior work on the psychoanalytic understanding of premenstrual syndrome (Hansen, 2014), I described the ways in which the physicality of the pregnant mother's body problematizes the notion of a discrete self. As such, the pregnant body offers a rich symbol concerning the fundamental uncertainty of our personal boundaries. According to theorists such as Kristeva (1982), it is precisely this blurring of boundaries that is so disturbing to us. Therefore, it is unsurprising that motherhood could be associated with psychosis, as the experience of motherhood might in itself be considered a "psychotic" one. Interestingly, in the developmental literature, motherhood, or "matrescence," is often unacknowledged as a significant developmental stage for women (Athan & Reel, 2015). Perhaps this is because the subjectivity of mothers does not correspond with current Western notions of "individuation" or healthy self-identity. In fact, maternal desire can be understood as quiet the opposite—the wish to blur one's identity, in essence, to lose one's boundaries to another. Conception and sex constitute yet other examples of the blurring of boundaries, as sperm, egg, and DNA, combine into an individual that is an amalgamation of two. Later, with pregnancy, the experience of confused boundaries becomes a physical one.[5] Post-birth, motherhood itself then becomes a further loss of boundaries as childcare requires a shift in individual subjectivity, so much so that British psychoanalyst Donald Winnicott once proclaimed "There is no such thing as a baby" (1947, p. 88). In sum, more attention needs to be paid to the ways in which "psychopathology" is understood, particularly as it overlaps greatly with women's healthy subjective experiences. Diagnosis is by its very nature inherently divisive, thus favoring this notion in the structure of its discourse. Further developing conceptualizations of both psychosis and maternal desire and how they relate to "self-disturbance" can provide insight into the post-partum experience.

PSYCHOANALYSIS

One of the earliest psychoanalytic accounts of postpartum psychosis was that of Gregory Zilboorg in 1928. Although Zilboorg uses strict Freudian terminology, he presents postpartum psychosis as a conflict between a rejection of traditional feminine roles and the occurrence of motherhood/pregnancy. In his theory, the birth of a child leaves the woman feeling punished and devoid of power (i.e., "castrated"), as a result, she "turns away, by the denial of reality or by a return to the masculine role" (p. 383). Here, postpartum psychosis is situated as occurring due to an adherence to cultural trends at the expense of an underlying unconscious striving to be in a more masculine role. Although couched within patriarchal language of early psychoanalysis, Zilboorg's theory can perhaps be considered an early feminist interpretation of the disorder.

More recently, the most direct and elaborate discussion of postpartum psychosis from within the greater psychosis literature can be found in Karon and Vandenbos's seminal book, *Psychotherapy of Schizophrenia: The Treatment of Choice.*[6] In a chapter by Rosenberg and Karon (1981), the authors review the then current literature on postpartum psychosis which stated that the psychological factors associated with postpartum psychosis were the physical discomfort of pregnancy (i.e., sleeplessness, pain, and physical exertion of delivery), the meaning of motherhood for the woman, and sexual guilt. They specifically reference Boyd, who believed that for many women, motherhood was equated with an end to their youth and an irrevocable tie to a husband they disliked. In terms of sexual guilt, Boyd hypothesized that some women may feel that pregnancy is punishment for sexual enjoyment. Rosenberg and Karon state that these hypotheses offer inadequate justification for why psychosis occurs postpartum, and appear to be more aligned with a neurotic presentation (i.e., anxiety or guilt symptoms). They highlight that most psychotic reactions occur after childbirth, suggesting that postpartum psychosis is the result of unconscious fantasies related directly to the traumatic nature of childbirth itself, rather than motherhood more generally. Specifically, the authors suggest that pregnancy is a gratification of oral fantasies, as the vagina "filled up" with semen is like the mouth filled up with milk. In this regard, childbirth is seen as a sudden, disastrous loss of this gratification. Rosenberg and Karon use a case study of a woman diagnosed with schizophrenia unremittent since childbirth to illustrate their conceptualization of postpartum psychosis. This case study, although certainly exemplary of their theory, also implicates maternal ambivalence in the maintenance of postpartum psychosis. For example, the woman portrays her psychological condition as the result of pregnancy, which she described as "going through the mill" (p. 331) and the result not of intercourse but a more hostile force whom she termed "the state" (p. 331). The patient stated ". . . my husband badgered me to marry him I accepted, thinking he would provide me with the things I needed, food and a home. When it turned out that he couldn't, I became pathological. The mill, or pregnancy as you call it, also did this and I got lockjaw" (p. 333). The therapist interpreted her "lockjaw" as a punishment for desiring oral gratification, to which the patient angrily said the therapist was as draining as all of her other interpersonal relationships. Notwithstanding this patient's need for oral gratification, her predicament can also be directly understood in relationship to social expectations of women in 1950s America. Her "lockjaw" may not be so much a punishment for wanting to suck from the breast or penis, as suggested by Rosenberg and Karon, but as a punishment for speaking against the societal demands that women get married in order to leave home, have children and put others' needs before their own.

In another earlier paper, Cohen (1968) analyzed a case of postpartum psychosis after an artificial insemination produced the birth of a female child. In this case, Cohen (1968) attributed postpartum psychosis to the artificial insemination, which activated Oedipal fantasies. The psychosis, which was conceptualized as brought about by guilt, included a regression into a fantasy in which the patient believed she was the Virgin Mary and had an Immaculate Conception. Cohen (1968) described this as a defensive retreat from her feelings of "dirtiness."

A third paper, by Roth (1975), recounts the case of a woman who experienced postpartum psychosis after a traumatic Caesarian birth. The woman re-experienced psychosis after her daughter birthed a child. The author explored the concept of "identity diffusion" in relationship to postpartum psychosis, seeing this diffusion resulting from the conflict in the mothering role of caring for a helpless and relatively noncommunicative infant. Roth (1975) also focused on the role of body image in postpartum psychosis, connecting the particular physiological state of motherhood to Freud's concept of the "bodily ego." In this light, postpartum psychosis is thought to arise from difficulty reintegrating the body image after birth of a child.

According to a Psychoanalytic Electronic Publishing (PEP) Web search conducted in October 2016, there have been no major psychoanalytic articles on postpartum psychosis published within the last forty years. This is particularly unfortunate given the large advances in psychoanalysis that have subsequently occurred, such as developments in attachment theory, greater feminist engagement within psychoanalytic scholarship, and a greater understanding of women's development across the lifespan (including situating motherhood as a developmental epoch).

SPIRITUALITY

One of the more neglected areas in the understanding of postpartum psychosis is the connection to spiritual concerns. Psychosis has long been recognized as having a spiritual dimension. Many people who experience psychosis remark on the religious or spiritual imagery that arises, often viewing psychosis as a form of "spiritual awakening" or "emergence." Jones, Kelly, Shattell, and Luhrmann (2016) discuss the ways in which many people with psychosis engage in "double booking-keeping" when providing explanatory models of their experiences, simultaneously understanding their experiences as supernatural or spiritual *and* as the result of a neuropsychological illness. Interestingly, motherhood too has been viewed by many as an opportunity for greater spiritual connection and awareness. Athan and Miller (2013) examine how motherhood in its various guises (e.g., adoption, stepmothering, birthing) brings women to experience a shift in perspective that aligns with world religions and other wisdom traditions. In their qualitative study on mothers' subjective experiences, Athan and Miller found six overlapping themes: 1) unconditional love and interdependence; 2) transcending ego or self-centeredness; 3) compassion and empathy; 4) mindfulness and heighted awareness; 5) meaning and purpose in life; and 6) faith in a higher power. Winnicott (1960) describes the early mother-child relationship as one of "magic" and not an "object relationship." In the case of women who have experienced traumatic birth histories, such as high-risk deliveries and perinatal loss, Athan, Chung, and Cohen (2015) found that many mother's conceptions of God included ideas regarding self-realization and learning through suffering. They state, "Suffering as a vehicle for knowledge of a spiritual reality has been the subject of most perennial wisdom traditions and may reflect these mothers own meaning-making processes of the complexities they faced" (p. 229). Taken together, this research suggests that spirituality may also be important for understanding postpartum psychosis. The connection between spiritual emergence, motherhood, and psychosis needs to be further articulated.

TREATMENT

Currently there are no specific psychological therapies or interventions for postpartum psychosis, either in its treatment or prevention. Treatment and prevention is currently centered exclusively on biomedical approaches. Electroconvulsive therapy (ECT) is a routinely-used treatment for postpartum psychosis (Babu, Thippeswamy, & Chandra, 2013). The use of ECT is primarily in the interests of the infant, as unlike antipsychotic medication, there is little risk toward the children of women who breastfeed. In a naturalistic prospective study of ECT use in India for postpartum psychosis, researchers found catatonic symptoms were significantly higher among women who received ECT than in those who did not (Babu et al., 2013). Doucet, Jones, Letourneau, Dennis, and Blackmore (2011) did a systematic review of interventions for the prevention and treatment of postpartum psychosis using database searches beginning with the year 1970. Their search found twenty-seven studies, ten focusing on prevention and seventeen on treatment. The study reported that preventative interventions were mood stabilizers, antipsychotic medications, and hormone therapy, and treatments for active postpartum psychosis as ECT, mood stabilizers, antipsychotics, hormones, and beta blockers. No psychological treatments or prevention methods were listed.

There are many barriers to the development of psychological treatments for postpartum psychosis. As mentioned previously in this chapter, a primary focus on biological etiology significantly curtails scholarship pertaining to psychological treatment and prevention methods. If postpartum psychosis is seen as primarily a biomedical phenomenon, then psychosocial approaches receive scant attention. Another possibility is that since postpartum psychosis has conceptually been associated with infanticide or infant risk, people may be quick to use medical interventions rather than psychological supports. That is, the infant's needs are considered as primary and may lead to the acceptance of more invasive procedures such as ECT. In addition, as psychosocial aspects of postpartum psychosis have not been adequately explored, we do not know exactly what the unique needs are for mothers experiencing postpartum psychosis, particularly with respect to how the infant should be incorporated into treatments. Many psychiatric facilities do not have mother-baby units, which may prevent the exploration of more holistic and dyadic psychosocial treatments. In addition, although for many women it may be the first time they have had a psychotic episode, mothers experiencing postpartum psychosis do not fit the standard image of a "first episode" psychosis client, thereby limiting their ability to access these types of services. Although some organizations, such as Action on Postpartum Psychosis in the United Kingdom, are promoting the use of Experts by Experience for peer support, this model has not typically been introduced in other countries, such as the United States. Clearly there is a great deal of work to be done regarding psychological approaches to the prevention and treatment of postpartum psychosis. Therapies that focus on all phases should be explored from acute onset to recovery. Researchers should work to tailor current psychosis therapies to the unique needs of mothers, including Cognitive-Behavioral Therapy for Psychosis (CBTp) and Mindfulness approaches. Peer support should be more strongly supported.

RECOVERY

The prognosis of women who have experienced postpartum psychosis is generally thought to be good. Most women recover spontaneously within a few months and return to normal social and occupational functioning. However, there is indication that some women who experience postpartum psychosis are at risk for developing puerperal and nonpuerperal psychotic episodes in the future. Estimates for future psychotic relapse rates are variable, with research listing 17–50 percent of cases for puerperal relapse and 39–81 percent for nonpuerperal relapse (Robertson & Lyns, 2003). However, much more information is needed about the psychosocial factors that contribute to both forms of relapse.

Women without reoccurring episodes may experience other difficulties. Robertson and Lyons (2003) state, "although the psychotic episodes ended for these women, they continue to live with the psychological after-effects for years" (p. 415). For example, many mothers are left with feelings of guilt, believing they have made others suffer during their psychosis. They may feel they did not pay adequate attention to their child during this time period and may fear that their psychosis may have impacted their child's emotional or intellectual functioning. In addition, they may also be concerned about what will happen with subsequent pregnancies. In Robertson and Lyons (2003) qualitative analysis of mothers' reports of postpartum psychosis, they found themes regarding feelings of loss of control—both of themselves and their treatment options. They also experienced a deterioration of their relationship with their partner and anger at the lack of knowledge of medical experts on postpartum psychosis.

In a qualitative study conducted in Sweden, researchers found that recovery was understood by some mothers as an intentional decision to return to health and daily life, as though having literally made the choice to get better (Engqvist & Nilsson, 2014). Many women in the study found a return to socializing a marker of recovery, particularly with other mothers. One mother in the study specifically noted that her recovery was predicated on the need to take time out for herself and not focus exclusively on her child. Many women described the need for social supports in terms of caring for their children and homes. In terms of psychological support, many of the women felt therapy was an immense help in their recovery. Importantly, therapy was not constrained to focusing on current circumstances, but also extended to reflecting on one's own childhood and their own experiences of being mothered. All the women in the study found medications helpful, but also found them to limit their ability to live life fully. Most women found recovery "really" happened when all medications were stopped.

CONCLUSION

The purpose of this chapter was to explore postpartum psychosis from multiple points of view, including the historical, social, psychoanalytic, and lived perspectives. The main aim was to provide a review of the literature through which to call for greater scholarship on postpartum psychosis from both feminist communities and progressive psychosis researchers. Although the majority of scientific and public discourse focuses on biological factors such as the rapid decline in oestrogen and progesterone levels following birth (Cookson, 1982) there are many social and psychological factors that need further exploration. In general, postpartum psychosis is an under-researched area. More attention needs to be paid to qualitative research, specifically on women's subjective experiences of postpartum psychosis, as well as on psychodynamic, spiritual perspectives, and socioeconomic and cultural contexts. It is anticipated that expanding discourse on postpartum psychosis will lead to the development of psychological treatment options for mother's experiencing this unique form of distress.

REFERENCES

Action on Postpartum Psychosis. (2014). Planning pregnancy: A guide for women at risk for postpartum psychosis. Birmingham, UK: Action on Postpartum Psychosis.

Agrawal, P., Bhatia, M. S., & Malik, S. C. (1990). Postpartum psychosis: a study of indoor cases in a general hospital psychiatric clinic. *Acta Psychiatr Scand, 81*(6), 571–75.

American Psychiatric Association. (2013). *Diagnostic and statistical manual of mental disorders* (5th ed.). Washington, DC: American Psychiatric Association.

American Psychiatric Association. (2000). *Diagnostic and statistical manual of mental disorders: DSM-IV-TR.* Washington, DC: American Psychiatric Association.

Athan, A. M., Chung, S., & Cohen, J. S. (2015). Spirtiual beliefs of mothers with potentially distressing pregnancies. *Spirituality in Clinical Practice. 2*(3): 216–32.

Athan, A. M., Klimowicz, A., Jobe, C.; Stewart, C., Wierzbinska, E., Muresan, T., Hoy, C. (Nov. 2013) "Where are Mothers?" (WAM)—a Systematic Review of Interdisciplinary Literature on Maternal Mental Health. Poster presented at the Perinatal Mental Health Meeting, Chicago.

Athan, A. M. & Miller, L. (2013). Motherhood has opportunity to learn spiritual values: Experiences and insights of new mothers. *Journal of Prenatal and Perinatal Psychology and Health*, 27(4), 220–53.

Athan, A. M. & Reel, H. L. (2015). Maternal psychology: Reflections on the 20th anniversary of Deconstructing Developmental Psychology. Feminism & Psychology, 25(3), 1–15.

Babu, G. N., Thippeswamy, H., & Chandra, P. S. (2013). Use of electroconvulsive therapy (ECT) in postpartum psychosis--a naturalistic prospective study. *Arch Womens Ment Health, 16*(3), 247–51. doi:10.1007/s00737-013-0342-2.

Benedetti, G. (1987). *Psychotherapy of schizophrenia.* London: Jason Aronson, Inc.

Bokhari, R., Bhatara, V. S., Bandettini, F., & McMillin, J. M. (1998). Postpartum psychosis and postpartum thyroiditis. *Psychoneuroendocrinology, 23*(6), 643–50.

Blackmore, E. R., Rubinow, D. R., O'Connor, T. G., Liu, X., Tang, W., Craddock, N., & Jones, I. (2013). Reproductive outcomes and risk of subsequent illness in women diagnosed with postpartum psychosis. *Bipolar Disorder, 15*(4), 394–404.

Blackmore, E. R., Jones, I., Doshi, M., Haque, S., Holder, R., Brockington, I., & Craddock, N. (2006). *British Journal of Psychiatry, 188*, 32–6.

Cohen, K. D. (1968). A case of postpartum psychosis following pregnancy by artificial insemination. *Psychoanalytic Quarterly,* 37:159.

Cookson, J. C. (1982). Post-partum mania, dopamine, and estrogens. *Lancet, 2*(8299), 672.

Doucet, S., Dennis, C. L., Letourneau, N., & Blackmore, E. R. (2009). Differentiation and clinical implications of postpartum depression and postpartum psychosis. *J Obstet Gynecol Neonatal Nurs, 38*(3), 269–79. doi:10.1111/j.1552-6909.2009.01019.x.

Doucet, S., Jones, I., Letourneau, N., Dennis, C. L., & Blackmore, E. R. (2011). Interventions for the prevention and treatment of postpartum psychosis: a systematic review. *Arch Womens Ment Health, 14*(2), 89–98. doi:10.1007/s00737-010-0199-6.

Ebeid, E., Nassif, N., & Sinha, P. (2010). Prenatal depression leading to postpartum psychosis. *J Obstet Gynaecol, 30*(5), 435-438. doi:10.3109/01443611003802321.

Engqvist, I., & Nilsson, K. (2014). The Recovery Process of Postpartum Psychosis from Both the Woman's and Next of Kin's Perspective—An Interview Study in Sweden. *Open Nurs J, 8*, 8–16. doi:10.2174/1874434601408010008.

Farkas, M. (2007). The vision of recovery today: what it is and what it means for services. *World Psychiatry, 6*(2), 68–74.

Focht, A., & Kellner, C. H. (2012). Electroconvulsive therapy (ECT) in the treatment of postpartum psychosis. *J ECT, 28*(1), 31–33. doi:10.1097/YCT.0b013e3182315aa8.

Gibson, L. E., Alloy, L. B., & Ellman, L. M. (2016). Trauma and the psychosis spectrum: A review of symptom specificity and explanatory mechanisms. *Clin Psychol Rev, 49*, 92–105. doi:10.1016/j.cpr.2016.08.003.

Gilman, S. L. (1976). *The face of madness: Hugh Diamond and the origin of psychiatric photography.* New York: Brunner/Mazel.

Grosz, E. (1994). *Volatile bodies: Toward a corporeal feminism.* Bloomington: Indiana University Press.

Halvorson, S. C. (2004). *Beth: A story of postpartum psychosis.* Bloomington, IN: Author.

Hansen, M. C., Vakhrusheva, J., Khan, S., Ramirez, P. M., & Kimhy, D. (2016, September). *Impact of the characteristics of auditory hallucinations on quality of life in people diagnosed with schizophrenia.* Poster presented at the International Consortium on Hallucination Research, Chicago, IL.

Hyman, R. (2004). Medea of suburbia: Andrea Yates, maternal infanticide, and the insanity defense. *Women's Studies Quarterly,* 32 (*3/4*), pp. 192–210.

Jaspers, K. (1923/1963). *General Psychopathology.* Chicago: University of Chicago Press.

Jones, I., & Craddock, N. (2001). Familiality of the puerperal trigger in bipolar disorder: results of a family study. *Am J Psychiatry, 158*(6), 913–17. doi:10.1176/appi.ajp.158.6.913.

Jones, I., & Smith, S. (2009). Puerperal psychosis: identifying and caring for women at risk. *Advances in Psychiatric Treatment, 15*(6), 411–18.

Jones, N., Kelly, T., & Shattell, M. (2016). God in the brain: Experiencing psychosis in the postsecular United States. *Transcult Psychiatry, 53*(4), 488–505. doi:10.1177/1363461516660902.

Jones, N., Kelly, T., Shattell, M., & Luhrman, T. (2016). "Did I push myself over the edge?": Complications of agency in psychosis onset an development. *Psychosis.* 8(*4*).DOI: 10.1080/17522439.2016.1150501.

Karraa, W. (2013, October 15). There are no words: Postpartum mood disorders and Miriam Carey's death | Psychology Benefits Society. Retrieved March 10, 2014, from http://psychologybenefits.org/2013/10/15/postpartum-mood-disorders/.

Kendell, R. E., Chalmers, J. C., & Platz, C. (1987). Epidemiology of puerperal psychoses. *Br J Psychiatry, 150*, 662–73.

Kisa, C., Aydemir, C., Kurt, A., Gulen, S., & Goka, E. (2007). [Long term follow-up of patients with postpartum psychosis]. *Turk Psikiyatri Derg, 18*(3), 223–30.

Klompenhouwer, J., van Hulst, A., Tulen, J., Jacobs, M., Jacobs, B., & Segers, F. (1995). The clinical features of postpartum psychoses. *Eur Psychiatry, 10*(7), 355–67. doi:10.1016/0924-9338(96)80337-3.

Kristeva, J. (1982). *Powers of horror: An essay on abjection.* New York: Columbia University Press.

Lieberman, J. A., Drake, R. E., Sederer, L. I., Belger, A., Keefe, R., Perkins, D., & Stroup, S. (2008). Science and recovery in schizophrenia. *Psychiatric Services, 59*(5): 487–96.

Lopez, O. V., Blanco, C., Keyes, K., Olfson, M., Grant, B., & Hasin, D.S. (2008). Psychiatric disorders in pregnant and postpartum women in the United States. *Arch Gen Psychiatry,* 65:805–15.

McCarthy-Jones, S. (2012). *Hearing voices: The histories, causes, and meanings of auditory verbal hallucinations.* New York: Cambridge University Press.

McWilliams, N. (2015). More simply human: on the universality of madness, *Psychosis, 7*(1), 63–71.

Moyer, J.H. (2014). *A mother's climb out of darkness: A story about overcoming postpartum psychosis.* Amarillo, Texas: Praeclarus Press, LLC.

Munk-Olsen, T., Laursen, T. M., Pedersen, C. B., Mors, O., & Mortensen, P. B. (2006). New parents and mental disorders: a population-based register study. *JAMA, 296*(21), 2582–589. doi:10.1001/jama.296.21.2582.

Nager, A., Johansson, L. M., & Sundquist, K. (2005). Are sociodemographic factors and year of delivery associated with hospital admission for postpartum psychosis? A study of 500,000 first-time mothers. *Acta Psychiatr Scand, 112*(1), 47–53. doi:10.1111/j.1600-0447.2005.00525.x.

Nager, A., Johansson, L. M., & Sundquist, K. (2006). Neighborhood socioeconomic environment and risk of postpartum psychosis. *Arch Womens Ment Health, 9*(2), 81–86. doi:10.1007/s00737-005-0107-7.

Nelson, B., Parnas, J., & Sass, L. A. (2014). Disturbance of minimal self (ipseity) in schizophrenia: clarification and current status. *Schizophr Bull, 40*(3), 479–82. doi:10.1093/schbul/sbu034.

Nelson, B., & Raballo, A. (2015). Basic self-disturbance in the schizophrenia spectrum: Taking stock and moving forward. *Psychopathology, 48*(5), 301–09. doi:10.1159/000437211.

Noll, R. (2000). *The encyclopedia of schizophrenia and other psychotic disorders.* New York, Facts On File, Inc.

Pescosolido, B. A., Martin, J. K., Long, J. S., Medina, T. R., Phelan, J. C., & Link, B. G. (2010). "A disease like any other"? A decade of change in public reactions to schizophrenia, depression, and alcohol dependence. *Am J Psychiatry, 167*(11), 1321–330. doi:10.1176/appi.ajp.2010.09121743.

Rashed, M. A. (2015). A critical perspective on second-order empathy in understanding psychopathology: phenomenology and ethics. *Theor Med Bioeth, 36*(2), 97–116. doi:10.1007/s11017-015-9323-y.

Rendon, C. (2013, October 4). Capitol Hill lockdown: Miriam Carey 'thought Obama was stalking her' and 'taking schizophrenia medication' | Mail Online. Retrieved March 10, 2014, from http://www.dailymail.co.uk/news/article-2442703/Capitol-Hill-lockdown-Miriam-Carey-thought-Obama-stalking-taking-schizophrenia-medication.html.

Rosberg, J. & Karon, B. P. (1981). A contribution to the understanding of postpartum psychosis. In B.P. Karon & G. R. Vandenbos (Eds.). *Psychotherapy of Schizophrenia: The Treatment of Choice,* pp. 329–37. New York: Jason Aronson.

Roberston, E., & Lyons, A. (2003). Living with puerperal psychosis: A qualitative analysis. *Psychology and Psychotherapy: Theory, Research and Practice,* 76: 411–31.

Roth, N. (1975). The mental content of puerperal psychoses. *American Journal of Psychotherapy,* 29(2): 204–11.

Schwartz, R. C., & Blankenship, D. M. (2014). Racial disparities in psychotic disorder diagnosis: A review of empirical literature. *World J Psychiatry, 4*(4), 133–40. doi:10.5498/wjp.v4.i4.133.

Sharma, V., & Mazmanian, D. (2014). The DSM-5 peripartum specifier: prospects and pitfalls. *Arch Womens Ment Health, 17*(2), 171–73. doi:10.1007/s00737-013-0406-3.

Sharma, V., Smith, A., & Khan, M. (2004). The relationship between duration of labour, time of delivery, and puerperal psychosis. *J Affect Disord, 83*(2-3), 215–20. doi:10.1016/j.jad.2004.04.014.

Showalter, E. (1987). *The Female Malady: Women, Madness, and English Culture 1830–1980.* Paris, France: Virago Press.

Spinelli, M.G. (Ed.) . (2002). *Infanticide: Psychosocial and legal perpsectives on mothers who kill.* Arlington, VA: American Psychiatric Publishing.

Thrailkill, J.F. (2002). Doctoring "The Yellow Wallpaper." *EHL, 69*(2), 525–66.

Tovino, S. A. (2010). Scientific understandings of postpartum illness: Improving health law and policy? *Harvard Journal of Law & Gender*, 3(31), 99–174.

Twomey, T.M. (2009). *Understanding Postpartum Psychosis: A Temporary Madness.* Westport, CT: Praeger.

Upadhyaya, S. K., Sharma, A., & Raval, C. M. (2014). Postpartum psychosis: risk factors identification. *N Am J Med Sci, 6*(6), 274–77. doi:10.4103/1947-2714.134373.

U.S. Census Bureau. (2014). Fertility of women in the United States. Retrieved from: https://www.census.gov/hhes/fertility/about/.

Ussher, J. M. (2006). *Managing the Monstrous Feminine: Regulating the Reproductive Body.* New York: Routledge.

Vassos, E., Pedersen, C. B., Murray, R. M., Collier, D. A., & Lewis, C. M. (2012). Meta-analysis of the association of urbanicity with schizophrenia. *Schizophr Bull, 38*(6), 1118–123. doi:10.1093/schbul/sbs096.

Weiser, M., Werbeloff, N., Vishna, T., Yoffe, R., Lubin, G., Shmushkevitch, M., & Davidson, M. (2008). Elaboration on immigration and risk for schizophrenia. *Psychol Med, 38*(8), 1113–119. doi:10.1017/S003329170700205X.

Werner, S., Malaspina, D., & Rabinowitz, J. (2007). Socieoeconomic status at birth is associated with risk of schizophrenia: Population-based multilevel study. *Schizophr Bull,33*(6), 1373–8.

Winnicot, D.W. (1960). The theory of the parent-infant relationship. *International Journal of Psycho-Analysis*, 41: 585–95.

Winnicot, D.W. (1947). *The Child, the Family, and the Outside World.* London: Penguin Books.

World Health Organization.(1992).*The ICD-10 Classification of Mental and Behavioural Disorders: Clinical Descriptions and Diagnostic Guidelines.* Geneva: World Health Organization.

Varner, L. (2002, April 16). The thousand stories of postpartum depression. *The Seattle Times.* Retrived from: http://community.seattletimes.nwsource.com/archive/?date=20020416&slug=lynne16.

Zilboorg, G. (1928). Post-partum schizophrenias. *Journal of Nervous & Mental Disease, 68*(4), 370–83.

NOTES

1. In comparing postpartum psychosis to postpartum depression, Ussher (2006) states, "Post-natal psychosis, a condition that affects less than 0.01 per cent of women giving birth, is a very different disorder, associated strongly with previous experience of psychosis and a biological predisposition to future psychotic episodes, with birth acting as a trigger" (p. 100).

2. The exact sentence reads: "Voices may occur shortly after a woman gives birth. These appear to be relatively rare, occurring after only 0.1 per cent of births" (p. 122).

3. A notable exception to this tendency is *Psychosis* journal, which actively promote collaborative, service-user, and psychiatric survivor research, as well as research that focuses on sociocultural, psychological, and subjective experiences of individuals. However, journals covering the subject with higher impact factor scores (e.g., *Schizophrenia Bulletin*) are less likely to include collaborative research and more likely to contain neurobiological and genetic research.

4. However, it is important as well to understand these prior diagnoses not just as indication of prior biological predisposition, but also within the context of a societal tendency to pathologize women's experiences, that may result in diagnoses such as "bipolar."

5. In fact, one can think of the heightened emotions on both sides of the abortion debate as unconscious attempts to separate mother from child.

6. At the time Rosenberg and Karon were writing, as today, there was confusion regarding the existence of postpartum psychosis as a distinctive category; that is, if pregnancy is the primary factor or if psychosis after childbirth occurs only in conjunction with an already underlying psychotic disorder.

Chapter Five

Disordered Eating and Distorted Thinking in Women

A Continuum in Objectification in Anorexia and Psychosis

Jessica Arenella

For nearly a century there have been reports of co-occurring eating disorders and psychosis but there has been little progress in understanding the relationship between the two. While research findings have been inconsistent regarding the co-occurrence of eating disorders and schizophrenia (Seeman, 2014), clinical observations have persisted for decades (i.e., Nicolle, 1936; Palazzoli, 1971; Robinson, 1973; Hugo & Lacey, 1998; Mavrogiorgou, Juckel & Bauer, 2001; and Seeman, 2016). When working with women presenting symptoms of psychosis, I too, have been struck by the incidence of eating disordered behaviors across people diagnosed with bipolar and schizophrenia spectrum disorders. Many women have reported the onset of psychosis following dieting and weight loss, while others have started to hear voices and develop delusional ideas related to compulsive eating and weight gain. Additionally, the link between psychosis and food control is found even in the absence of a clinical eating disorder. Dieting, food restriction, and weight loss have been observed to precipitate psychotic episodes in people with and without a prior history of psychiatric illnesses (Robinson & Winnik, 1973; Jiang et al., 2006).

This chapter will focus on intrapsychic (occuring within the mind), interpersonal, and socio-cultural models to address the overlapping psychological factors in disordered eating and psychosis. Given the substantial changes in diagnostic criteria for eating and psychotic disorders over time, I will focus on symptomatology rather than the presence of any particular psychiatric diagnosis. I will outline a psychodynamic hypothesis, using the ideas of Arieti (1974), Palazzioli (1971), and Searles (1965), for understanding the possible relationships between disordered eating and psychosis, as mediated by trauma and women's experience in Western culture. Specifically, I will argue that disordered eating and psychosis both involve concretization and externalization of intrapsychic and socio-cultural conflicts that result in structural changes in the psyche, although to varying degrees.

The relationships between disordered eating and psychosis is often complicated by iatrogenic factors in both weight loss and psychosis. For example, weight loss medications, often amphetamine derivatives, can provoke psychosis, as in the case of a woman I worked with[1] who was given these drugs in her adolescence and went on to have a lifetime of manic and depressive episodes. Subsequent dieting, without pharmacological agents, often triggered recurrence of her manic and psychotic episodes. Antipsychotic and hypnotic medications also tend to stimulate appetite, night eating, and weight gain, which may elicit compensatory behaviors. While the atypical antipsychotics are notorious for inducing metabolic changes that lead to weight gain, studies of patients with anorexia treated with these drugs show they do not gain weight (Lebow, Sim, Erwin, & Murad, 2012). This may be due to noncompliance with the medication or other eating-disordered behaviors to avoid this side effect. To date, there are no medication treatments for disordered eating with a robust evidence base (Frank & Shott, 2016).

As early as 1913, there were clinical reports of women who developed psychosis following a period of dieting (Nicolle, 1936). At one time it was even suggested that anorexia was a "pre-psychotic" condition, as it involved the "fanatical domination of one idea" (Nicolle, 1936, p. 153) namely, to starve oneself. Stretching beyond the strictly intrapsychic model, and interpreting disordered eating practices through the lens of contemporary gender norms, Nicolle suggested that, for a young woman whose future is bound up with attracting the right man, control over her bodily appearance and weight are the few spheres of power that she possesses. More recently, there has been a shift toward viewing the distorted body image and logical fallacies found in disordered eating as psychotic or pseudo-psychotic symptoms to be treated with antipsychotic medications. Lebow, Sim, Erwin, and Murad (2013) explain that "the irrational cognitions" in anorexia are similar to delusions insofar as they are ego-syntonic and are not amenable to insight even when the person's life is potentially at risk. Hearing voices, depersonalization, derealization, rigidity of thought, and over-valued ideas can also be found in both disordered eating and psychosis (Seaman, 2014). Poor attachment, social isolation, and poor treatment alliance and adherence have also been suggested to be similarities (Seaman, 2014). These overlapping features continue to be a source of interest and exploration, even if the presence of full-blown disordered eating and diagnoses of schizophrenia or schizoaffective disorder do not necessarily overlap in a statistically significant manner.

A recent Norwegian study prospectively examined the self-reported psychiatric symptoms of a sample of over 11,000 fifteen- and sixteen-year-olds (Bratlien et al., 2013). They found that adolescents who went on to develop psychotic disorders were more likely to report anxiety, depression, and "feeling in need of treatment for eating disorders" (p. 221). Similarly, in an Italian study of over 700 high school girls, researchers found that both anorectic and bulimic patients were more likely than controls to endorse the idea that "something is wrong with your mind," a common item on many psychosis measures (Miotto et al., 2010, p. 240). Additionally, the patients diagnosed with anorexia were more likely to report that they never feel close with other people and the patients diagnosed with bulimia were more likely to report that others are to blame for their problems. While these beliefs are not psychotic, they are indicative of the withdrawal, isolation, and externalization of threat that characterize psychosis.

Studies of intrusive mental images in psychological disorders have demonstrated the relative frequency of such mechanisms in disordered eating, psychosis, and post-traumatic stress disorder (Brewin, Gregory, Lipton & Burgess, 2010; Cili & Stopa, 2015). These involuntary, persistent, vivid, distressing, and detailed images may be one of the neural mechanisms that contribute to the formation of dis-ease in people whose bodily integrity has been compromised through childhood maltreatment (Brewin et al., 2010). The images of a heavy, bloated, permeable, unprotected, or injured body may in turn trigger unhealthy eating behaviors.

There have also been studies of what has been termed the "anorexic voice" (Tierney & Fox, 2010, p. 243); a critical, merciless, self-monitoring commentary on one's eating behavior that can also issue restrictive commands (see Pugh and Waller, 2016). In her memoir about her eating disorder, Caroline Knapp (2003) explained that she heard the anorexic voice as a "hiss of self-recrimination" (p. 10) triggered by eating too much, being too ambitious, or over-desiring sexual contact. This voice would speak the phrase: "You're a pig, a sloth, you suck" (p. 10). She also shared the experience of a friend who hears the similarly-worded phrase "You're a pig, you're a fucking, fucking fat pig" (p. 85) when she feels her pants are tight. A client I have been working with also hears the frequent refrain as "Pig, pig," especially when she walks by younger and more slender women.

There are remarkable similarities between self-reports of the "anorexic voice" and the voices that are experienced in the context of psychosis. Tierney and Fox (2010), in a thematic analysis of interviews with thirty-seven women with eating disorders, delineated three stages in the development of the anorexic voice. The first stage begins when, during a period of stress or vulnerability, a voice emerges that is seen as a friendly companion and a helpful coach who sorts out the confusion and gives some clear advice. During the second stage, the woman is drawn into the relationship with the voice, which begins to be perceived as a relentless tyrant who hijacks the woman's daily life. The third stage is achieved in recovery, when the woman mourns the loss of her unpleasant yet constant companion and develops a life without the anorexic voice.

The voices experienced in the context labelled psychosis also generally begin during period of stress or vulnerability (Romme & Escher, 1993). The voice may be supportive or antagonizing, or there may be a combination of both positive and negative voices (Romme & Escher, 1993). As with anorexic voice, the perceived power imbalance (i.e., the voice is negatively valanced and seen as more powerful than the person) is a marker of functional impairment (Pugh & Waller, 2016; Rosen et al., 2015; Tierney & Fox, 2010). This is often when a person comes to the attention of the mental health system and is diagnosed with a psychotic disorder. However, recovery in psychosis may or may not include elimination of voices. Many voice-hearers find recovery in achieving a more equitable balance of power between the voice hearer and the voices (Romme, Escher, & Dillon, 2009), and the voices may continue lifelong.

Seeman (2014) has found inconsistent research data regarding the co-morbidity of diagnosed eating disorders and psychosis. While the incidence of psychosis is rarely noted in populations of eating disordered patients, eating disorders are found among patients diagnosed with psychosis at a higher rate than the general population (Seeman, 2014). The reasons for this discrepancy are unclear but Seeman (2014) suggests that it may have to do with patterns of treatment-seeking, and that psychotic disorders are more likely to arouse the need for treatment, while eating disorders often go undetected for many years.

In an attempt to make sense of the various permutations of co-occurring eating disorder behaviors and psychosis in her clinical practice, Seeman (2014) formulated seven hypotheses for their possible relationship. She proposes: 1) eating disorders and psychoses are separate disorders that occur together by chance; 2) that eating disorders are a prodrome for psychosis (or vice-versa, that psychotic symptoms can be an early sign of an eating disorder); 3) eating disorders are a form of psychosis involving delusional beliefs; 4) transient psychosis occurs in people whose metabolic and electrolyte imbalance are disturbed by a primary eating disorder; 5) psychotic symptoms occur in a subset of more severe cases of eating disorders; 6) medications used for treating eating disorders can trigger psychosis and those used for psychosis can trigger eating disorders; and 7) controlling food intake is a means of obtaining positive self-efficacy for individuals who feel that they are at risk of psychotic disintegration. Seeman (2014) tests these hypotheses reviewing available literature and finds that there is some evidence for all of these hypotheses, yet none is conclusive.

Previous clinical and research literature, however, has given scant attention to a common factor in the development of eating disorders and psychosis—child abuse is a common antecedent to both of these conditions. The recent meta-analysis by Caslini et al. (2016), concluded that childhood physical, sexual, and emotional abuse are significantly correlated with bulimia nervosa and binge eating disorder, while the link between abuse and anorexia nervosa remains inconclusive. According to a 2012 meta-analysis in *Schizophrenia Bulletin*, Varese et al. (2012) found that adverse childhood events, including sexual, physical, and emotional abuse, are prominent risk factors for psychosis, with a nearly three-to-one odds ratio. From a research perspective alone, the mediating factor of childhood abuse seems a promising area to explore. In addition, the psychological and emotional sequelae of childhood abuse may also be a predisposing factor in the development of psychosis and disordered eating. Interpersonal trauma in childhood can lead to difficulties in establishing secure attachment and lead to further trauma from having conflicted or absent relationships (Arenella, 2001; Herman, 1992; NCTSN, n.d.). Difficulty in regulating emotions and overuse of problematic approaches to self-regulation, such as dissociation, engaging in high-risk behaviors, substance abuse, and acting out, may also stem from childhood abuse (Herman, 1992; NCTSN, n.d.). These common responses to trauma may contribute to the unease, inadequacy, shame, guilt, confusion, and despair that can crystallize into disordered eating or psychotic "solutions" (Jen, Saunders, Ornstein, Kamali & McInnis, 2013).

Psychodynamic theory provides a fruitful model to approach the relationships between childhood trauma and the development of psychiatric symptoms (Arenella, 2000). While much psychiatric literature focuses on a few narrow symptoms of a particular diagnostic iteration, psychodynamic theory provides a means to organize the wide variety of psychological, physiological, and behavioral sequelae of child abuse. Psychodynamic theory was founded in part to address the very problem of premature physiological stimulation and the aftermath of trauma. Ferenczi (1955) suggested that childhood sexual and physical abuse contributed to the development of ego fragmentation and dissociative defenses. This is particularly important given that fragmentation and dissociation are common features of psychotic experience (Moskowitz, Schafer & Morahy, 2008).

Psychodynamic theory places a strong emphasis on the role of childhood physiological changes and experiences in the development of personality. Bodily experiences and how they are managed by the child and adult are considered the cornerstone of psychological development. Anzieu (1989) and others (see Arenella, 2000 for details) have suggested that skin sensations experienced with regularity over time facilitate feelings of boundedness and independence from other animate and inanimate objects. When infants develop the motor skills to interact in more complex ways with their bodies and the world, their perspectives on reality can become more sophisticated. The ego is hypothesized to emerge out of a need to mediate between bodily sensations and the demands of reality. Not surprisingly, the original elaboration of the body ego centered on the male experience but later authors focused on the role of the female body in the development of the woman's body ego (Barnett, 1966; Bernstein, 1983, 1993; Keiser, 1954; Kleeman, 1976; Silverman, 1981). Given the nature of female genitalia as less clearly bounded and not fully visible, it has been suggested that disruption in the healthy development of the body ego would heighten the abused girl's concern for bodily integrity, specifically regarding access, penetrability, and diffusivity (Arenella, 2000).

While I do not find it fruitful to conceptualize disordered eating attitudes as psychotic *per se*, there are parallels that are significant and may help elucidate the persistent riddle of these problematic expressions of severe psychic distress. The threat of physical, psychological, or emotional destruction that occurs in childhood distress predisposes some individuals toward extreme and stubborn cognitive and behavioral alterations. Disordered eating and psychosis both involve a dramatic narrowing and externalization of anxiety, often at the expense of other areas of functioning, especially the interpersonal. The drive to escape the painful constraints of human dependence by disavowing one's subjective needs can lead toward a mechanistic objectification of oneself.

Not surprisingly, there has been considerable feminist analysis of eating disorders, focusing on the intense scrutiny of the female body, the increasing media pressure to conform to an idealized figure, internalized sexism, and other sequelae of patriarchy. While some feminists view the anorexic body as a rejection of an oppressive feminine ideal, others see anorexia as the outcome of excessive conformity to the ubiquitous directive for women to lose weight and maintain a slender body at all costs. Knapp (2003) described her experience of decimating the female body in her memoir of anorexia: "I stopped menstruating. I had no breasts. The body was tight, taught, bolted down. It did not curve or bulge or protrude, it did not bleed" (p. 183). Yet, she also writes about the constant self-monitoring and comparing that many women perform around food and weight: "Tiny slices [of cake], no frosting, forty-five minutes on the Stairmaster: These are the conditions, variations on a theme of vigilance and self-restraint that I've watched women dance to all my life . . . the knee jerk measuring of self against other: . . . [W]ho's thin, who's fat, how do I compare?" (Knapp, 2003, p. 25).

Bordo (1993) and Chernin (1985) suggest that anorexia, most profoundly, expresses ambivalence about carrying out the female role by simultaneously rejecting the reproductive capacity and embracing the cultural dictate to diet.

The woman with anorexia is at once compliant and defiant. Interestingly, Arieti (1974) describes a similar contradiction in the schizoid[2] child who later develops psychosis. He writes that such children may appear to be very compliant but that the compliance is superficial and that, "In order to avoid anxiety, he becomes a person uncommitted to what he is doing or what he is participating in" (Arieti, 1974, p. 104). He concludes that, "the schizoid reaches a pseudo solution by denying a great part of his life, but by doing so he may make the part of this life that he continues to live more awkward and unstable" (Arieti, 1974, p. 105).

Anorexia may be interpreted psychodynamically as a way for the person to combat her own shame at needing connection and sustenance. She may attempt to shield the vulnerable self by defensively revoking her own desire for anything at all. In her memoir, Hornbacher (1998) describes eating disorders as, "a bundle of deadly contradictions: a desire for power that strips you of all power. A gesture of strength that divests you of all strength. A wish to prove that you need nothing, that you have no human hungers, which turns on itself and becomes a searing need for the hunger itself" (p. 10). Knapp (2003) writes of the overt and covert messages to women about their hunger, their desire: "Don't eat too much, don't get too big, don't reach too far, don't climb too high, don't want too much. No no no" (p. 11). She fears that she is "so hungry, [she]'ll never get fed" (Knapp, 2003, p. 9). These misogynist cultural dicta offered a solution to Knapp's anxiety and insecurity: "At a time when I felt adrift and confused and deeply unsure of myself, starving gave me a goal, a way to . . . exert control, something I could be good at" (Knapp, 2003, p. 9).

The shame and sensitivity of the woman engaging in disordered eating to her own needs and desires may—paradoxically—lead to the self-imposed denial of need. Arieti (1974) writes of an analogous development in the pre-psychotic person whose sensitivity, especially to perceived hostility, is so intense that he or she withdraws altogether. He explains that, "a common defense among schizoid persons is that of decreasing their needs to an almost unbelievable extent" (p. 111). For example, one of my clients who has suffered with psychosis and disordered eating described giving or throwing away all of her belongings and sleeping on the wooden floor of her apartment during the early stage of one of her breakdowns. Later, she hitchhiked barefoot across the country and lived in a convent.

Recently, Mitropoulos et al. (2015) analyzed the manifest content of male and female symptoms in in-patients diagnosed with psychosis and found significant gender differences. Nearly 16 percent of a sample of women with psychosis described delusions related to accusations of, or forced, sexual immorality. For example, these women reported hearing voices calling them "slut," "whore," and "prostitute" and had delusions related to pornography and being impregnated by injection. The authors interpret this data in terms of the role of societal prescriptions of gender in the expression of psychosis. Given the high rate of childhood abuse, including sexual abuse, among women diagnosed with psychosis, it is important to consider that these themes may reflect shame regarding real sexual abuse. These themes are also consistent with the schizoid and eating-disordered ambivalence regarding desire. Knapp (2003) explains that the story of her anorexia is also about, "the guilt that's aroused when a woman tests old and deeply entrenched rules about gender and feminism. It's about the collision between self and culture, female desire unleashed in a world that's still deeply ambivalent about female power and that manages to whet appetite and shame it in equal measure" (p. 19).

In Arieti's account of the development of psychosis, he describes a prodromal phase of "pre-psychotic panic." This is a period of intense but vague anxiety. He describes its feeling as if one were in a "jungle" where the threats are ideas about feeling "unwanted, unloved, unlovable, [. . .] inadequate, unacceptable," and "unable to find his way, [. . .] discriminated against, suspected" (Arieti, 1974, p. 120). Arieti notes that the "jungle" that is experienced during the pre-psychotic panic is in part created by a society that can be competitive and cruel, favoring brutishness over sensitivity and compassion, a society that does indeed exclude nonconforming and nonsuave[3] individuals. However, he notes that the "jungle" is also a psychic state created by the patient's own anguish and uncomfortable vulnerability and the person's own poor sense of self that colors her view of others.

In her memoir, Knapp (2003) writes that, following a disappointment and abandonment by a boyfriend, she decided, "'Okay, I'll just stop eating.' The sentence just popped into my head, fully formed and non-negotiable. A solution: I am overwhelmed (by need, by disappointment, by uncertainty) and this is how I'm going to react" (p. 48). This type of reductionistic switch is a key concept underlying Arieti's theory of psychosis. He writes that psychosis emerges when "the indefinite feelings become finite, the imperceptible becomes perceptible, the vague menace is transformed into a specific threat" (Arieti, 1974, p. 123). While not delusional *per se*, the emergence of the solution of disordered eating represents a similar abrupt narrowing of the focus of anxiety. Arieti explains that once the person passes from this phase of pre-psychotic anxiety into true psychosis, the intense but vague sense of hostility and threat is transformed into a specific and externalized threat. The person is no longer subject to crippling low self-esteem because she or he has become the target of an unfair, malevolent, and relentless persecutor. The painful self-reproach for myriad shortcomings is replaced by a concrete and specific threat in the outside world.

For Arieti, psychosis is marked by a structural alteration in the psyche. While the conflictual themes and distorted ideation have personal meaning for understanding the individual undergoing a psychotic break, it is the breakdown in the formal processes of thinking that defines psychosis. When dysfunctional family dynamics present as hallucinatory voices, psychosis is present. The content helps the clinician understand the dynamic conflicts that have preceded the psychosis, but it is the form that these conflicts take that constitute psychosis. He refers to the "perceptualization of the concept" (Arieti, 1974, p. 268) as the transformation from the overwhelming and disturbing emotional conflicts into persecuting voices, malodors, violating sensations, and nightmarish visions. Although these unusual perceptions can be understood metaphorically, for the person laboring under the influence of psychosis these perceptions are experienced as concrete reality.

Drawing heavily on the work of Palazzoli, Arieti (1974) opines that in anorexia the body is "blamed" in "another instance of concretization," (p. 330) a concept similar to how conflicts are thought to be concretized in schizophrenia. She hypothesizes that the psyche withdraws from both the complexity and the pain of anxiety in an effort to forestall further emotional damage; and the interpersonal, intrapsychic, and social conflicts are reduced to preoccupation with the body. Palazzioli (1971) suggests that for the person with an eating disorder, "the body is felt as a threatening entity that must not be brutally destroyed, but must merely be held in check" (p. 201). She argues that the woman with anorexic behaviors, "experiences food intake as an enhancement of her body at the expense of herself" (Palazzioli, 1971, p.201).

When the fear of one's body becomes paramount, avoidance of food intake may be understood as an effort to keep this threatening entity (i.e., the body) as small and contained as possible. Part of the concretization of the body in disordered eating involves viewing one's body as a thing, a bad object. Paradoxically, the fight against being a thing takes place at the level of thingness and therefore grows more desperate but can never be won (Palazzioli, 1974). The woman engaged in anorexic behaviors perhaps preemptively objectifies herself rather than be objectified by society at large. In treating herself as an object, she may hope to subdue what otherwise may be subject to ridicule, abuse or disappointment.

When considering the objectification of women, it is crucial to return to a wider socio-cultural lens. Searles's paper, "The Effort to Drive the Other Person Crazy," describes the family dynamics that contribute to confusions about reality in individuals with psychosis; however, his observations can also be applicable to broader sociocultural dynamics. He explains that interpersonal interactions that stimulate emotional conflict by arousing different parts of oneself in opposition to each other are likely to provoke madness. For instance, a client of mine once shared that, while studying abroad with her esteemed opera teacher, the teacher's attractive spouse tried to initiate an affair with her and she was torn between desire to please her teacher and desire to lose her virginity. Closely related, Searles (1965) suggests that interacting with a person upon two or more "quite unrelated levels of relatedness simultaneously" (p. 258), as well as rapid switching back and forth between levels of relatedness, can also be maddening. An example of this might be a parent who is sexually abusing a child, and alternates between behaving as a regular parent and exploiting the child for his or her own sexually sadistic needs.

One need not look too far to see how the widespread, contradictory messages to women about our bodies and gender roles might be considered crazy-making. While women have made unprecedented advances in education, sports, jobs, and financial and political power in the United States, there are also unprecedented expectations of women to manage their bodies. Hair removal has expanded from face, legs, and underarms, to complete pubic hair removal. Not only are eyes lifted and tummys tucked but "vaginal rejuvenation" and labioplasty are on the rise. The cultural prescriptions for women's bodies have become even more detailed and unattainable. In a stunning (or, perhaps, cynical) paradox, the very women's fashion, beauty, and fitness magazines that create, promote and inundate women with blueprints for our bodies have commented on how unattainable these expectations are. For example, a recent article in *Harper's Bazaar* noted that, "none of the body trends over the past few decades have felt as head-scratchingly inaccessible for the average woman lacking a trust fund-size budget for personal trainers, diet coaches and plastic surgeons as the current ideal: D-cup breasts, tiny waists, sculpted abs, big butts and thigh gaps inches-wide—all in one" (Tunnell, 2015, June 19).

Shape magazine promotes the use of the hashtag #LOVEMYBODY alongside articles on how to get "flat sexy abs" in ten minutes. While the United States was on the verge of electing its first female presidential candidate from a major party in 2016, millions of young women were being subjected to unprecedented scrutiny of their bodies.

These irreconcilable communications—to love one's body and to change it, to be a powerful woman and to micromanage all of one's body parts so as not to offend the patriarchy—surely contribute to the impossibility of womanhood and likely influence the expression of one's individual psychic struggles. Hornbacher (1998) writes of her own experience with an eating disorder, "I chose an eating disorder. I cannot help but think that, had I lived in a culture where "thinness" was not regarded as a strange state of grace, I might have sought out another means of attaining that grace," (pp. 6–7). Furthermore, it may be that the dieting and preoccupation with body size are more socially acceptable for women and provide a language for those struggling with the double-bind of modern womanhood. In my observation and experience, these conflicting communications to women play a role in the expression of eating disorders and also a legion of subclinical patterns of disordered eating.

The enduring kinship between disordered eating and psychosis may be found in the structural changes in the psyche that take place, likely in response to childhood trauma. While the trauma may be in the form of overt adverse childhood experiences, it may also take place in poisonous but not abusive interactions. The overwhelming threats to self are split off and externalized so that they can be quarantined. For those with disordered eating, the body becomes the captive enemy, closely constricted in an attempt to protect the vulnerable self. In psychosis, while the body may or may not be perceived as problematic, nonetheless, the chaos and terror within is firmly placed into the outside world, separate from the self. This externalization is simultaneous with a radical narrowing of concern, such that battling the enemy is prioritized over one's own physical well-being. While the symptoms of psychosis and disordered eating serve to protect, they also further isolate the struggling and traumatized person. The presence of voices may serve to ameliorate the social isolation and encourage chronicity by keeping the person attached to a problematic way of living.

Perhaps it is because conflicts are played out in the realm of the concrete and external that the expressions of these disorders become a mirror of our own cultural psychopathology.

Medical anthropologists and historians have found that the expression of various symptoms change over time and place in so far as they reflect the symbols and values of the era. When comparing the content of voices ("auditory hallucinations") across cultures, Americans tend to experience more violent and aggressive messages, and there is some evidence that violent voices may be on the rise over the past few decades (Larøi et al., 2014). This suggests that voices may reflect the concerns and conflict not only of the individual, but of the society as a whole. Similarly, in more communal societies, the voices of ancestors are more prevalent, where as in more individualistic societies, there are more alien or mechanistic voices reported (Luhrmann, Padmavati, Tharoor and Osei, 2015).

Given the unprecedented deluge of increasingly detailed (and distorted) media images of women's bodies, combined with rapid changes in women's roles in society, it is not surprising that eating issues would take on psychotic proportions. While we learn a great deal about the madness of our society in the symptomatic expression of disordered eating and psychotic patients, we must remember that those who are suffering are not choosing their form of protest against society, but are putting into sharp relief, at much detriment to themselves, the pathology of our culture and time.

REFERENCES

ANRED—Anorexia & Eating Disorders Information and Resources. (n.d.). Retrieved July 12, 2016, from http://www.anred.com/stats.html.

Anzieu, D. (1989). *The Skin Ego*. (Chris Turner, Trans.) New Haven: Yale University Press.

Arenella, J. (2000). Rorschach indicators of body image disruption and precocious maturity in sexually and physically abused girls (Doctoral dissertation, Long Island University). (UMI No. 9959123).

Arieti, S. (1974). *Interpretation of Schizophrenia*. New York: Basic Books.

Barnett, M. C. (1966). Vaginal awareness in the infancy and childhood of girls. *Journal of the American Psychoanalytic Society, 14*, 129–41.

Bernstein, D. (1983). The female superego: A different perspective. *International Journal of Psychoanalysis, 64*, 187–201.

Bernstein, D., Freedman, N., & Distler, B. (1993). *Female Identity Conflict in Clinical Practice*. Northvale, NJ: Jason Aronson.

Bordo, S. (1993). *Unbearable Weight: Feminism, Western Culture, and the Body*. Berkeley: University of California Press.

Bratlien, U., Øie, M., Haug, E., Møller, P., Andreassen, O. A., Lien, L., & Melle, I. (2013). Self-reported symptoms and health service use in adolescence in persons who later develop psychotic disorders: A prospective case-control study. *Early Intervention in Psychiatry, 9*(3), 221–27. doi:10.1111/eip.12102.

Bremser, J. A., & Gallup, G. G. (2012). From one extreme to the other: Negative evaluation anxiety and disordered Eating as candidates for the extreme female brain. *Evolutionary Psychology, 10*(3). doi:10.1177/147470491201000306.

Brosnan, M., Ashen, C., Walker, I., & Donahue, J. (2010, October). Can an 'Extreme Female Brain' be characterised in terms of psychosis? *Personality and Individual Differences. Personality and Individual Differences, 49*(7), 738–42.

Caslini, M., Bartoli, F., Crocamo, C., Dakanalis, A., Clerici, M., & Carrà, G. (2016). Disentangling the association between child abuse and eating disorders. *Psychosomatic Medicine, 78*(1), 79–90. doi:10.1097/psy.0000000000000233.

Chernin, K. (1985). *The Hungry Self: Women, Eating and Identity*. New York: Times Books.

Effects of Complex Trauma. (n.d.). Retrieved July 23, 2016, from http://www.nctsn.org/trauma-types/complex-trauma/effects-of-complex-trauma.

Farber, S. K. (2008). Autistic and dissociative features in eating disorders and self-mutilation [Abstract]. *Modern Psychoanalysis, 33*(1), 23–49.

Ferenczi, S. (1955). Confusion of tongues between adults and the child: The language of tenderness and passion (E. Mosbacher, Trans.). In M. Balint (Ed.), *Final Contributions to the Problems and Methods of Psycho-analysis* (pp. 157–67). London: Hogarth Press. Original work published in 1933.

Frank, G. K., & Shott, M. E. (2016). The role of psychotropic medications in the management of anorexia nervosa: Rationale, evidence and future prospects. *CNS Drugs, 30*(5), 419–42. doi:10.1007/s40263-016-0335-6.

Götestam, K. G., Eriksen, L., & Hagen, H. (1995). An epidemiological study of eating disorders in Norwegian psychiatric institutions. *International Journal of Eating Disorders, 18*(3), 263–68. doi:10.1002/1098-108x(199511)18:33.0.co;2-o.

Herman, J. L. (1992). *Trauma and recovery*. New York: BasicBooks.

Hornbacher, M. (1998). *Wasted: A memoir of anorexia and bulimia*. New York: Harper Collins.

Hospers, H. J., & Jansen, A. (2005). Why homosexuality is a risk factor for eating disorders in males. *Journal of Social and Clinical Psychology, 24*(8), 1188–201. doi:10.1521/jscp.2005.24.8.1188.

Hudson, J. I., Pope, H. G., & Jonas, J. M. (1984). Psychosis in anorexia nervosa and bulimia. *The British Journal of Psychiatry, 145*(4), 420–23. doi:10.1192/bjp.145.4.420.

Hugo, P. J., & Lacey, J. H. (1998). Disordered eating: A defense against psychosis? *International Journal of Eating Disorders, 24*(3), 329–33. doi:10.1002/(sici)1098-108x(199811)24:33.0.co;2-r.

Jen, A., Saunders, E. F., Ornstein, R. M., Kamali, M., & Mcinnis, M. G. (2013). Impulsivity, anxiety, and alcohol misuse in bipolar disorder comorbid with eating disorders. *International Journal of Bipolar Disorders, 1*(1), 13. doi:10.1186/2194-7511-1-13.

Jiang, W., Gagliardi, J. P., Raj, Y. P., Silvertooth, E. J., Christopher, E. J., & Krishnan, K. R. (2006). Acute psychotic disorder after gastric bypass surgery: Differential diagnosis and treatment. *American Journal of Psychiatry, 163*(1), 15–19. doi:10.1176/appi.ajp.163.1.15.

Kadish, Y. A. (2012). Pathological organizations and psychic retreats in eating disorders. *The Psychoanalytic Review, 99*(2), 227–52. doi:10.1521/prev.2012.99.2.227.

Keeney, R., Smith, L., Sekoff, L., & Le, T. D. (2012, December 15). Gendered Diseases: How have autism and schizophrenia become engendered as the extreme male and female brains? Retrieved July 12, 2016, from https://prezi.com/hy8bxn6atdza/gendered-diseases/?utm_campaign=share&utm_medium=copy.

Keiser, S. (1954). Female sexuality. *Journal of the American Psychoanalytic Association, 4,* 563–74.

Kleeman, J. A. (1976). Freud's view on early female sexuality in light of direct child observation. *Journal of the American Psychoanalytic Association, 24,* supp. 5, 3–27.

Laroi, F., Luhrmann, T. M., Bell, V., Christian, W. A., Deshpande, S., Fernyhough, C., Jenkins, J, &Woods, A. (2014). Culture and hallucinations: Overview and future directions. *Schizophrenia Bulletin, 40*(Suppl 4). doi:10.1093/schbul/sbu012.

Lebow, J., Sim, L. A., Erwin, P. J., & Murad, M. H. (2012). The effect of atypical antipsychotic medications in individuals with anorexia nervosa: A systematic review and meta-analysis. *International Journal of Eating Disorders, 46*(4), 332–39. doi:10.1002/eat.22059.

Luhrmann, T. M., R. Padmavati, H. Tharoor and A. Osei (2015). Differences in voice-hearing experiences of people with psychosis in the USA, India and Ghana: Interview-based study. *British Journal of Psychiatry, 206* (1) 41–44; DOI: 10.1192/bjp.bp.113.139048.

Mavrogiorgou, P., Juckel, G., & Bauer, M. (2001, May). Recurrence of paranoid hallucinatory psychoses after beginning a fasting period in a patient with anorexia nervosa [Abstract]. *Fortschr itte der Neurol ogie- Psychiatr ie , 69*(5), 211–14. doi:10.1055/s-2001-13932.

Miotto, P., Pollini, B., Restaneo, A., Favaretto, G., Sisti, D., Rocchi, M. B., & Preti, A. (2010). Symptoms of psychosis in anorexia and bulimia nervosa. *Psychiatry Research, 175*(3), 237–43. doi:10.1016/j.psychres.2009.03.011.

Mitrani, J. (2007). Bodily centered protections in adolescence: An extension of the work of Frances Tustin [Abstract]. *International Journal of Psychoanalysis, 88*(5), 1153–1170. doi:10.1516/ijpa.2007.1153.

Mitropoulos, G. B., Gorgoli, D., Houlis, D., Korompili, K., Lagiou, C., & Gerontas, A. (2015). Psychosis and societal prescriptions of gender; a study of 174 inpatients. *Psychosis, 7*(4), 324–35. doi:10.1080/17522439.2015.1020333.

Moskowitz, A., Schäfer, I., & Dorahy, M. J. (2008). *Psychosis, trauma and dissociation: Emerging perspectives on severe psychopathology.* Chichester, UK: Wiley-Blackwell.

Nicolle, G. (1938). Pre psychotic anorexia. *The Lancet, 2,* 1173–1174.

Palazzoli, M. S. (1971). Anorexia nervosa. In S. Arieti (Ed.), *The World Biennial of Psychiatry and Psychotherapy* (Vol. 1, pp. 197–218). New York: Basic Books.

Pugh, M., & Waller, G. (2016). The anorexic voice and severity of eating pathology in anorexia nervosa. *International Journal of Eating Disorders, 49*(6), 622–25. doi:10.1002/eat.22499.

Robinson, S., & Winnik, H. Z. (1973). Severe psychotic disturbances following crash diet weight loss. *Archives of General Psychiatry, 29*(4), 559. doi:10.1001/archpsyc.1973.04200040099016.

Romme, M. & Escher, S. (Eds). (1993) *Accepting Voices.* London: MIND.

Romme, M., Escher, S., & Dillon, J. (2009). *50 Stories of Recovery.* Manchester: PCCS Books.

Rosen, C., Jones, N., Chase, K. A., Grossman, L. S., Gin, H., & Sharma, R. P. (2015). Self, voices and embodiment. *Journal of Schizophrenia Research, 2*(1), 1008. Retrieved from http://www.ncbi.nlm.nih.gov/pmc/articles/PMC4834921/.

Sabo, A.N. & Havens, L. (Eds.) (2000). *The Real World Guide to Psychotherapy Practice.* Boston: Harvard University Press.

Searles, H. F. (1965). *Collected Papers on Schizophrenia and Related Subjects.* New York: International Universities Press.

Seeman, M. V. (2014). Eating disorders and psychosis: Seven hypotheses. *World Journal of Psychiatry, 4*(4), 112. doi:10.5498/wjp.v4.i4.112.

Seeman, M. V. (2016, April 29). Eating disorders and psychosis. *Psychiatric Times, 33*(4). Retrieved   from   http://www.psychiatrictimes.com/special-reports/eating-disorders-and-psychosis.

Silverman, M. A. (1981). Cognitive development and female psychology. *Journal of the American Psychoanalytic Association, 29*, 581–605.

Tierney, S., & Fox, J. R. (2010). Living with the anorexic voice: A thematic analysis. *Psychology and Psychotherapy: Theory, Research and Practice, 83*(3), 243–54. doi:10.1348/147608309x480172.

Tunnell, A. (2015, June 19). The 2015 body is more unattainable than ever. Retrieved July 23, 2016, from http://www.harpersbazaar.com/beauty/diet-fitness/a11239/the-new-body-ideal/.

Unknown, R., & Sèchehaye, M. (1951). *Autobiography of a schizophrenic girl* (G. Rubin-Rabson, Trans.). New York: Grune & Stratton.

Varese, F., Smeets, F., Drukker, M., Lieverse, R., Lataster, T., Viechtbauer, W., Read, J, vanOs, J. & Bentall, R. P. (2012). Childhood adversities increase the risk of psychosis: A meta-analysis of patient-control, prospective- and cross-sectional cohort studies. *Schizophrenia Bulletin, 38*(4), 661–71. doi:10.1093/schbul/sbs050.

III

WOMEN, PSYCHOSIS & SPIRITUALITY

Chapter Six

Mystics, Witches, or Hysterics?

The Therapeutic Stakes When Spirituality Becomes a Symptom

Liane F. Carlson

In 1876, a woman approached the Belgian village of Bois-d'Haine on foot. She was only thirty-three, but in the photographs from the time she looks older, with deep lines drawing her full face downward and hints of grey starting to twist her dark hair into wiry spirals. She must have looked even more tired and disreputable than usual that day. She had arrived from Paris the evening before and spent the night beneath a tree. In the weeks she had spent plodding the 170 miles from the French capital to the small Belgian town, we know she had been stopped at least once but not much else about her journey. A doctor had found her in a tavern, half a litre into a bottle of beer "with people of even looser reputation than she" (cited in Hustvedt, 2011, p. 277), as he wrote in a letter back to Paris, when the reason for her journey struck. She began to convulse, her stomach swelled, and she started offering delirious arguments to anyone who listened from six in the evening until one in the morning. Versed in the latest medical knowledge of the day, the doctor ruled out pregnancy and instead held her down and pressed her ovaries until the attack ended. When she came to, she gave her name as Geneviève L., thanked him but declined any further help, explaining she was on her way to see "her sister Louise Lateau" in Belgium (Hustvedt, 2011, p. 278).

Geneviève L. was Geneviève Basile Legrande, a poor woman born out of wedlock, shuttled from foster family to foster family until an attack of hysteria at sixteen began the first of her many institutionalizations. In the years before her pilgrimage to Bois-d'Haine, she had lived a scattered life, bearing and giving up for adoption two illegitimate children who she dreamed of supporting as a seamstress during her periods of relative stability. At the time the village doctor found her, she was in between hospitalizations but still a frequent patient of Jean-Martin Charcot at Salpêtrière in Paris, where she was prized for the peculiarly religious nature of her symptoms. During any given attack, Geneviève might see demons, talk with Jesus, fall into trance-like prayer, hallucinate erotic caresses, refuse to eat, endure freezing temperatures without complaint, or lacerate her flesh.

The woman Geneviève was seeking was Louise Lateau, an individual with one of the best documented cases of the stigmata. Ever since 1868, when she was eighteen, blood would begin flowing punctually every Thursday night from her feet, hands, left side, and her heart. And every Friday night the wounds would vanish and Lateau would return to her work to support her family. In the hours between the start and stop of the stigmata, much like Geneviève, Lateau would fall into an ecstatic trance, insensible to pain and distraction as she witnessed the crucifixion. Physicians, priests, and pious pilgrims flocked to her, alternately eager to discredit her, investigate her for canonization, and venerate her.

Geneviève was hardly the only one to note the similarity between the pair. When the doctor who stopped her convulsions reached the point in his story where Geneviève related her plan to visit her "her sister Louise Lateau," he added the wry note, "as she called her, not without reason" (Hustvedt, 2011, p. 278). One of Geneviève's doctors at Salpêtrière, Désiré-Magloire Bourneville, went even further, writing an entire book arguing that Lateau was a hysteric, no different from the women like Geneviève he treated (Bourneville, 1878).

No different—except one was venerated by awestruck pilgrims and one was regularly mocked, assaulted, and brutalized, even by the medical staff assigned to treat her. Whatever the doctors or Geneviève herself thought of the connection that day, the villagers who guarded the entrance to Lateau's house did not see it. When she asked to see the stigmatic, they mocked her and turned her away. Heartbroken, she began the long trek back to Paris.

The image of the two women in that village, one despised as an outcast, one venerated as a saint, captures with unusual starkness a debate playing out across continents from the early years of the nineteenth century to today. What is the relationships between the sick woman and the saint? Does God really grant visions to select women or are they simply unbalanced, suffering from delusions that took on a pious shape favored by their society? If the visions of women like Geneviève could be explained as hysteria, what did that mean for the great women, like Teresa of Ávila or Catherine of Siena who had reported similar visitations? Could it be that the great spiritual mystics of past centuries had been suffering from some form of undiagnosed mental illness?

Complicating these questions is the fact that the doctors of Genevieve's day did not use contemporary terms, such as "schizophrenia" or psychosis. Rather, they diagnosed Geneviève with hysteria, a disease largely discredited today.

While this fact poses certain difficulties in interpreting her record, it also offers an unusual opportunity to examine the struggles between psychiatry and religion with relative disinterest. Freed from the need to defend a diagnosis, I want to spend this chapter exploring the relationship between psychosis, religion, and hysteria in Geneviève's day, with particular attention to the way preexisting religious and medical beliefs about women's bodies influenced the clinical diagnosis of hysteria in nineteenth century France. Far from breaking with tradition by equating female mysticism with hysteria, I argue, Geneviève's doctors were in fact continuing a long tradition of male authority figures legitimizing or delegitimizing the spiritual experiences of women, often with implicit, albeit hostile, sanction of the Catholic Church. In the final section, I want to turn from historical conversations and ask a normative question—namely, did the medical interpretation of her symptoms ease or exacerbate her suffering? And if it exacerbated her suffering, did her interpretation of her own life as one of pious suffering offer a form of escape from an overbearing medical establishment or ultimately confirm her doctors' arguments that religious ecstasy was hysteria by another name?

PSYCHOSIS, HYSTERIA, AND RELIGION IN CONTEXT

What do I mean by psychosis and how might Geneviève's case trouble current understandings of the term? Can we use contemporary terms of psychosis when talking about her diagnosis? What is at stake—and for whom—in medicalizing Geneviève's visions of God? These are some of the questions I will address in the following section, but before delving into the scientific, theological, and political debates that shaped Geneviève's diagnosis during her lifetime, I want to begin by offering a provisional definition of psychosis for the purpose of this chapter. When I speak of psychosis as a contemporary category, I am drawing on both the common, dictionary definition and the clinical definition in the fifth edition of the *Diagnostic and Statistical Manual of Mental Disorders* (*DSM-5*). According the *DSM-5*, psychotic and schizophrenic disorders are characterised by five symptoms: "delusions, hallucinations, disorganized thinking (speech), grossly disorganized or abnormal motor behavior (including catatonia), and negative symptoms" (American Psychiatric Association, 2013). The Oxford English Dictionary offers, in turn, a less formal definition of psychosis as, "a severe mental disorder in which thought and emotions are so impaired that contact is lost with external reality" (Psychosis, n.d). For my purposes, then, when I

use the word psychosis I am referring primarily to a mental disorder characterised by visions, hallucinations, and loss of contact with immediate, shared
reality.

However psychosis is defined, Geneviève would appear to present a clear
case of it by modern standards, at least on the surface. Her first extended stay
in a hospital for psychological treatment came at the age of fourteen. Until
that point, she had spent her life shuttled from foster family to foster family.
Finally, though, she had a burst of good fortune and found love with a young
man named Camille. The two became engaged and, for a brief moment,
Geneviève was genuinely happy. Soon, though, Camille died and the young
Geneviève was left desolate. Her foster father forbade her to go to his funeral
but the young Geneviève escaped. Distraught, she tried to throw herself on
his grave but was stopped by the other mourners. She collapsed and fell into
a prolonged depression. When her foster mother died shortly thereafter, her
foster father decided he could not handle the depressed, erratic, occasionally
violent young woman and returned her to the hospice in Poitiers, where
Geneviève spent a year undergoing hydrotherapy to cure her depression
(Hustvedt, 2011, p. 227–33).

That, at least, was the story Geneviève told her doctors. While her doctors
never doubted the veracity of her story, some doubt remains whether Camille
ever existed. Asti Hustvedt recounts hunting down all of the burial registers
near Geneviève's town between 1856 and 1858 but being unable to find
anyone named Camille except for a baby who died at twenty months. She
acknowledges that Camille might have come from a different town but also
hypothesizes that perhaps Camille never existed and was a phantom she
created to symbolize the constant abandonments of her youth (Hustvedt,
2011, p. 228).

Real or not, Camille figured hugely in Geneviève's mental life and visions in following years. Following her release from the hospital, she began
having visions and "hysterical episodes." During these fits, she would alternately flail, assume pious poses of prayer, proposition doctors for sex, and
speak to invisible presences. The two great themes of these episodes, which
would be termed psychotic today, were religion and her love for Camille. As
part of a recurring hallucination, Geneviève later told her doctors of an affair
she was having with a doctor who was really her dead lover Camille returned
from the grave (Hustvedt, 2011, p. 261–68).

Over 140 years have passed since Geneviève's time in Salpêtrière, making it difficult to parse how much of her reported biography was real and how
much was hallucinated. Did Camille exist? Is it possible she was having a
sexual relationship with an unscrupulous doctor? It is difficult to say for sure.
Regardless, it seems clear that Geneviève was subject to visions and periods
where she lost control of her motor skills, hallucinated the presence of the
dead, and was overwhelmed by feelings of religious ecstasy and lust. Yet I

want to argue in this section that, for all of the apparent similarities between Geneviève's case and the clinical definition of psychotic symptoms, labelling her as psychotic would be a deeply problematic move for both philosophical and historical reasons.

Philosophically, calling Geneviève's ecstatic visions of God hallucinations is a normative claim. It presupposes a shared commitment to a certain model of health, psychological stability, and integration into society as the highest good. As such, the diagnosis of psychosis also takes for granted that her visions were pathological, and that her doctors were right in understanding her visions as a loss of contact with reality, rather than a new form of contact with a different, higher reality. More to the point, the label of psychosis assumes that psychiatry is right to diagnose experiences previously considered religious, because psychiatry offers a "better" explanatory paradigm than religion. As one scholar summed up the problem with both approaches, assuming that spiritual and psychotic can be explained by the same psychological mechanisms "appear[s] to exclude God a priori as a causative agent and therefore exclude what the subject would regard as the key feature of his experience. Phenomenological approaches try to use clinical categories to explain the relationship between spiritual experience and psychopathology, but presuppose rather than explain the distinction" (Marzanski and Bratton, 2002, p. 360).

The implications of pathologizing visions of God are not merely troubling for the religious; even psychiatry struggles with the normative commitments implicit in the categories of spiritual experience and psychosis. In the late 1990s and the early 2000s, an article called "Spiritual Experience and Psychopathology" by Mike Jackson and K. W. M. Fulford initiated a series of exchanges in psychiatric journals about the boundaries between psychopathology and spiritual experience. Fulford and Jackson opened their article by noting phenomenological similarities between psychosis and spiritual experience, such as "time distortion, synesthesias, loss of self-object boundaries and the transition from a state of conflict and anxiety to one of sudden "understanding"' (Fulford and Jackson, 1997, p. 42). After noting the difficulties of defining spiritual experience and psychosis, neither of which had widely accepted meanings, they attempted to differentiate between the two by way of reflection on case studies. Spiritual experience, they concluded, differed from psychosis in that subjects positively evaluated their experiences, based on their own personal, spiritual values, and were able to function at higher level in their everyday lives because of their spiritual encounters (Fulford and Jackson, 1997, p. 54). Reactions to these criteria varied, from criticisms that Fulford and Jackson needed a stronger definition of spirituality that took into account the role of institutions in authenticating spiritual experiences (Marzanski and Bratton, 200, p. 316), to arguments insisting that canonical spiritual experiences within the Christian tradition have often been felt to be deeply distressing (Marzanski and Bratton, 2002, p. 366), to suggestions that the word "psychotic" is so overburdened with value judgments that it ought to be jettisoned altogether in favor of a more neutral term like "anomalous experiences" (Brett, 2002, p. 377). In sum, the boundaries between psychosis and religious experience are still in question today, even for those working in the field of psychiatry.

The difficulty of drawing sharp distinctions between psychosis and religious experience in Geneviève's case grows even sharper once placed in historical context. Some of those problems are specific to Geneviève's case. Her records are at times fragmentary, leaving long periods between her visits unaccounted for and simple facts about her life unverified. Her symptoms were observed through the filter of a largely defunct medical diagnosis, hysteria. As a result, questions that would have been highly interesting to a psychologist working even a few decades later—namely, was her second child a product of rape?—were never asked, while speculations about the nature of her parentage were pursued by doctors who believed in the hereditary nature of criminality. In addition to speculating about her past, her doctors also editorialized, comparing her behavior to demonic possession of the victims of medieval witch hunts. Their interest in making connections between her symptoms and religious beliefs was so explicit that her biographer Hustvedt (2011) felt obligated to verify that Geneviève's doctors had not fabricated that fact that she was born in Loudon, the site of a famous fifteenth-century possession. The doctors were reporting the truth in this instance, but Hustvedt's suspicions indicate the extent to which even Geneviève's medical records were not merely neutral records but, rather, entangled with a broader political battle against the Catholic Church. In short, the evidence is incomplete, slanted to reinforce the idea that her visions were psychotic, not spiritual, possibly embellished at points, and missing key facts.

If psychosis really is a value judgment that presupposes agreement on the origin and nature of visions, and if Geneviève's record really is compromised because of the context in which it is written, do we have to abandon altogether the question of how psychosis and religious experience relate in her life? I would suggest not. Instead, I want to argue that Geneviève's case provides a particularly interesting opportunity to examine attitudes toward religion during the birth of early psychiatric categories. To do so, I want to bracket the terminology of psychosis for the moment and discuss the psychiatric term used to diagnose Geneviève during her lifetime: hysteria, as defined by the director of Salpêtrière, Jean-Martin Charcot. By doing so, I am not abandoning the question of psychosis, as many classically psychotic symptoms like hallucinations were folded into the diagnosis of hysteria, so much as recontextualizing psychotic, religious symptoms as the site of conflict between early psychiatry, the Catholic Church, and the nascent field of religious studies, as each attempted to offer its own interpretive framework for the type of experience Geneviève represented.

At the center of this struggle was Jean-Martin Charcot. Born in 1825 to a middle-class Parisian family, Charcot distinguished himself early on for his brilliance as a medical student and would later rise to fame as "the father of neurology." After passing his medical examinations, he completed his internship at Salpêtrière. At the time, Salpêtrière was less a hospital, in our contemporary sense, than a holding pen for socially marginalized women. Beggars, vagabonds, epileptics, prostitutes, the disabled, and women suffering from venereal diseases were confined alongside the demented and those deemed to be suffering from incurable madness. Organization was minimal, cure rates low, and death rates high. In 1862, the year Charcot entered the hospital, there was only one doctor for every five hundred patients. Women were fed either once a day, twice a day, or put on a starvation diet (Didi-Huberman, 2003, p. 13). Only 9.72 percent of patients were declared cured. Meanwhile, officials ascribed 254 deaths to "causes presumed due to insanity," though the proximate causes of death recorded included "masturbation, scrofula, blows and wounds, debauchery and licentiousness, cholera, erotomania, alcoholism, rape . . . love, joy, "bad reading habits," nostalgia and misery' (Didi-Huberman, 2003, p. 15). Charcot himself called it, 'the great emporium of human misery' but vowed to return (Cited in Didi-Huberman, 2003, p.17).

Charcot got his wish and spent the rest of his career teaching and researching at Salpêtrière. He rose steadily to fame throughout his career, giving immensely popular public lectures, discovering over fifteen new diseases, and receiving the title "Professor of Pathological Anatomy" in 1872, followed by the "Clinical Chair of the Diseases of the Nervous System" in 1881. Charcot, who possessed a genuine gift for creating typologies of symptoms, was initially drawn to the hospital by the prospect of bringing order and understanding to the various forms of mental illnesses before him—all mental illnesses, not just hysteria. In fact, it was something of a bureaucratic accident that put Charcot in charge of the hysteria ward. No one really knew what to do with hysterics at the time. Their symptoms were maddeningly inconsistent. Some had seizures, some suffered partial paralysis, some grew mute, some grew deaf, some forgot their native language, some had visions, some spontaneously bled or physically mimicked the signs of pregnancy right up to hysterical childbirth. And some, like Geneviève, fell into religious ecstasies. One of the only traits they did seem to share did not seem particularly helpful for narrowing down the parameters of the disease: they were highly susceptible to suggestion.

Faced with an indiscriminate mixture of symptoms, Charcot sought to discover patterns that would help him categorize the progression of hysteria as a physiological disease. He was convinced that hysteria was real and a biological disease, caused by some sort of lesion on the brain. As a biological disease, he reasoned, it should follow regular, observable stages, like Parkinson's or Charcot's tooth or any of the other illnesses he had created diagnostic criteria for during his career. Charcot found those stages for what he called "grand hysteria," or at least he thought he did. In the first stage, the hysteric had convulsions that looked like epileptic seizures. In the second stage, she suffered from "clownism," or exaggerated contortions that mimicked circus performers. Next, she moved into "passionate poses," acting out feelings of terror or ecstasy. Finally, she ended by collapsing into delirium (Hustvedt, 2011, p. 21–22).

One of the noteworthy things about Charcot's diagnostic criteria is how visual they are—a point that will be germane later in this chapter. None of the four stages require the patient to speak or explain her experiences of a hysterical episode to a doctor. Note that even the diagnosis of the patient experiencing ecstasy or terror relied on observing the patient, not asking her if she felt terror. This emphasis on the visual led Charcot to prize photography, and later paintings, as uniquely precise ways of capturing a hysterical episode. In later years, he even went so far as to write books interpreting various paintings of the possessed in the history of art according to his four stages of hysteria (Hustvedt, 2011, p. 286).

His publications on hysteria and ecstasy in art were part of a broader struggle against supernatural, religious explanations for the behavior of women like Geneviève. As he described the project and hopes of the burgeoning science of neurology:

> While recognising that living beings present *phenomena that cannot be found in dead nature* [*nature morte*], and which therefore belongs to them alone, the new physiology *absolutely refuses* to see life as a mysterious and supernatural influence, which acts as fancy takes it, free from all laws. Physiology goes so far as to believe that vital properties will one day be reduced to properties of a physical order (cited in Didi-Huberman, 2003, p. 21).

Charcot was largely too diplomatic, or perhaps prudent, to take such sentiments to their logical conclusion and openly challenge religious authorities that might champion "mysterious and supernatural influences" as a form of causal explanation. Nevertheless, some of the doctors working under him, most noticeably Désiré-Magloire Bourneville, did wage that battle, presumably with Charcot's tacit permission. As noted earlier, Bourneville wrote a book on Louise Lateau, arguing that Lateau, like the saints before her, was a hysteric, no different from patients like Geneviève. He also demanded, successfully, that the nuns who served as hospital nurses be replaced with trained members of the laity (Goetz, Bonduelle, and Gelfand, 1995, p. 277).

The Catholic Church, for its part, pushed back by prompting the government to curb the growing field of neurology. The government, which associated anti-clericalism with republicanism, was happy to oblige (Goetz, Bonduelle, and Gelfand, 1995, p. 276). Charcot's students were denied doctoral degrees when their dissertations came across as too atheistic, and his lectures were cancelled when authorities determined they were too scientific (Hustvedt, 2011, p. 236). Charcot himself was branded an atheist by many Catholic doctors (Kugelmann, 2011, p. 38). The problem, as the Church saw it, was not merely that Charcot threatened their authority by undermining the credibility of their saints, though that was naturally part of the issue. Rather, the problem was also that Charcot advocated radical new therapeutic techniques like hypnosis. As Kugelmann (2001) argues, Catholics were particularly wary of hypnosis because it carried the aura of Spiritualism. Moreover, hypnosis required subjects to relinquish their wills to their hypnotizer. For clergy and laity, it was unclear whether the self-loss attending hypnosis should be viewed as harmless, or a pernicious, supernatural form of influence (Kugelmann, 2011).

Yet couching the relationship between Charcot and the Catholic Church as one of simple opposition misses key nuances. To begin with, some contemporary Catholic clergy were willing to recognize the link between hysteria and mysticism, at least within limits. In 1883 a Belgian Jesuit named Father Hahn published a book arguing that Saint Teresa of Ávila, one of the few female doctors of the Church, had been a hysteric. Hahn's book was later banned and he was forced to recant, but the mere publication of it hints at some degree of disagreement within the Catholic Church (Mazzoni, 1996, p. 37). Other Catholics and clergy members, though not willing to go quite so far as to label Teresa hysterical, were perfectly willing to admit that not all apparent miracles were genuine. Dr. Lefebvre, a Belgian doctor who taught at the Catholic University of Louvain, began his 1873 book analyzing Louise Lateau in medical terms by remarking,

> I shall perhaps astonish many readers by speaking in this way, if they are unacquainted with the traditions of the Catholic Church. In the world a twofold prejudice prevails. Some imagine that the Church is incessantly seeking after new revelations and miracles; others think that she is too slow nowadays in affirming facts of the supernatural order to our sceptical and scoffing generation. Both parties know little of the Church. Truth is heaven-born: whenever it descends to man, whether it be amidst popular applause, or whether it be lowly and despised, the Church, its Divine guardian, always receives it, always welcomes it with affection and respect. On the other hand, she has nothing to do with apocryphal miracles or with suspicious marvels; she feels no attraction towards error. Whenever she meets with it, masked though it be under the semblance of religion, she denounces it calmly but mercilessly (Lefebvre, 1873, p. 2).

Another Catholic contemporary of Charcot made the point more pithily when he drily observed about the reports of miraculous healing at Lourdes,

"A man who should declare the numberless cures of nervous maladies at Lourdes to be all of them due to our Lady's wonder-working power, may be a pious enthusiast, but is neither a prudent man nor a trustworthy advocate of the cause he is defending" (cited in Kugelmann, 2011, p. 149).

As these texts evidence, the Catholic Church felt its credibility was at stake in its confrontation with this radical new realm of medicine. It was hardly about to accept the suggestions of either Bourneville or Father Hahn that its most popular saints had been hysterics like the lower-class women who filled the wards of Salpêtrière. However, it was not above accepting that nervous maladies did exist and could be cured by suggestion. The struggle was not so much over the theory of hysteria as its scope and proposed cures.

Out of the struggle between Salpêtrière's efforts to demystify mysticism and the Catholic Church's maneuvers to limit the diagnosis of hysteria, a third interpretive framework was arguably emerging that treated religion as an object of scientific, scholarly study. The field of religious studies, as opposed to theology, is a relatively recent one that often dates itself back to anthropological work in the nineteenth century. There is a wealth of scholarship in the field today arguing that the great thinkers of the nineteenth century did more than just invent a new way of thinking about religion; they actively invented religion as a category. As these texts argue, many of the traditions considered world religions today, such as Judaism and Hinduism, lacked the word "religion" or the idea of it as a sphere separate from everyday life and ritual (Batnitzky, 2011; Nongbri, 2013). In practice, European elites consolidated religion as a distinct object of knowledge by defining it in contrast to the practice of other, usually disenfranchised, minority groups. At times, these definitions grew out of a self-interested desire to limit the power of theocracies. Such was the case when the excommunicated Jewish philosopher Baruch Spinoza contrasted superstition with true religion based in faith in God, justice, and charity (Spinoza, 2006, p. 1). At other times, however, the distinction between true religion and superstition or barbarism was made by missionaries or colonial officials in positions of power who used the indigenous population's putative lack of religion as justification for their paternalistic rule (Masuzawa, 2005; Chidester, 1996).

In effect, these thinkers were policing what counted as genuine religious experience and what was superstition. By calling women like Geneviève hysterical rather than pious, the doctors at Salpêtrière were participating in this broader European conversation about what counts as acceptable forms of religious expression. Not coincidentally, two of the canonical figures within religious studies, Émile Durkheim and Sigmund Freud, attended Charcot's lectures on hysteria. Diagnosing hysteria, then, was about far more than accurately interpreting a set of baffling symptoms. It was in a very real way part of a broader struggle to consolidate new disciplines and old authority structures by staking out the right to define what counted as "true" religion.

But what led these various institutions to choose hysteria and a woman like Geneviève—obscure, socially marginalized and in no way a figure of social veneration—as the site of that struggle? The answer to that question lies in contemporary beliefs about women. In the next section I want to suggest that it was not a mere accident of fate that led so many different interpretations and institutions to cluster around the figure of the hysteric. Rather, it was the history of thinking about hysteria as a woman's problem grounded in biological weakness and in need of male interpretation that led figures like Charcot and Bourneville to treat Geneviève's symptoms as a stand-in for religious experience more generally.

WOMEN AND PSYCHOSIS

For Charcot, Bourneville and the rest of the doctors working at Salpêtrière in the latter half of the nineteenth century were hardly the first to notice the strange overlap between religious experience and strange, seemingly un-caused symptoms in women. Instead, I want to argue in the following pages that their equation of bodily malady and female spirituality simultaneously follows a long medical tradition of understanding hysteria as a woman's disease borne out of the peculiar vulnerability of the female body and a Christian tradition of prioritizing certain, visual, somatic signs of women's spirituality.

Hysteria, as Georges Didi-Huberman phrased it "was the symptom . . . of being a woman" (Didi-Huberman, 2003, p. 68). The very names given to the condition attest to the long history of diagnosing hysteria as a woman's condition. Etymologically, the word "hysteria" derives from the Greek word for "womb," "hystera." Other names circulated in France, as well, ranging from the neutral-sounding appellations of "spasms, nerve aches, vapors," to phrases that suggested the origin of the disease in abstinence, such as "mel-ancholia of virgins and widows," to names that explicitly reiterated the link between hysteria and the uterus, such as "uterine suffocation, womb suffoca-tion . . . 'suffocation of the mother' . . . uterine epilepsy, uterine strangula-tion, uterine vapors, and uterine neurosis" (Cited in Didi-Huberman, 2003, p. 69).

The theories explaining hysteria were equally clear about the link be-tween female biology and the disorder. Early Hippocratic texts suggested that, "The womb is the origin of all diseases" in women (Scull, 2009, p. 13). Other writers in Ancient Greece working in the Hippocratic tradition pushed the connection further, hypothesizing that the uterus was an animal that "wandered" in the abdomen. As writers such as Celsus and Aretaeus sug-gested, when the uterus pressed against organs such as the lungs or throat, it produced experiences of choking, paralysis, and shortness of breath (Scull,

2009, p. 12). Other thinkers, such as Galen (129 CE–c. 200/c. 216), argued that hysteria resulted from sexual abstinence and recommended marriage as a cure. Still others, including Plato in some readings, straddled both theories, describing the uterus as, "a living creature with a desire for childbearing" which would become "vexed and aggrieved" if left unfertilized for too long and take to wandering through the body (Adair, 1996, p. 154).

The idea that a wandering womb gave rise to hysteria persisted for centuries. As late as 1681, the English physician Thomas Willis argued against received wisdom when he wrote, "the body of the womb is of so small a bulk, in virgins and widows, and is so strictly tyed by the neighbouring parts round about, that it cannot of it self be moved, or ascend from its place, nor could its motion be felt if there were any" (cited in Scull, 2009, p. 31). Willis, like Charcot after him, preferred to locate hysteria in disorders of the nervous system.

Nervous disorders were not as obviously tied to female biology as uterine disorders but soon collided with pre-existing beliefs about the greater sensibility of women. Women were often seen as more porous and impressionable than men. As Elaine Showalter argues, "In the eighteenth century, there was a gender split in the representation of the body, with the nervous system seen as feminine, and the musculature as masculine" (Showalter, 1993, p. 293). Even when men displayed stereotypical symptoms of hysteria, they were often diagnosed with "neurasthenia," a nearly identical disorder attributed to intellectual overexertion, rather than emotional lability. For a brief period, being diagnosed as a neurasthenic even served as a mark of distinction for men. It was considered a disease of the elite. In time, though, that privileged passed and neurasthenia became associated with women who diverted their physical energy from the task of childbirth to intellectual competition with men (Showalter, 1993, p. 297).

Many of these beliefs about the greater sensitivity of the female nervous system were still espoused when Charcot wrote. A contemporary of Charcot's, Pierre Bricquet, made the point explicitly in an 1859 text that explained hysteria as a disease of impressions and affective sensations. "The woman," Bricquet wrote, "in order to fulfil her providential mission, must present this susceptibility to a much greater degree than man" (cited in Didi-Huberman, 2003, p. 73). To his credit, Charcot did not fall into the trap of thinking about hysteria as solely a woman's disease. On the contrary, he was proud of the small ward for male hysterics he had developed, correctly noting that he was one of the few people researching male hysteria (Showalter, 1993, p. 309).

For all of his relatively progressive attitudes about the link between sex and hysteria, when Charcot conducted his lectures in Salpêtrière he was nevertheless intervening in a long history that understood hysteria as a set of symptoms rooted in female biology. This history was by no means independent of religious interpretations of women's visions. However much the doctors at Salpêtrière occasionally liked to position themselves as breaking from a barbaric past that condemned sick women to the stake, the truth is that the idea that authority figures only began medicalizing mysticism in the nineteenth century is a fiction. Even in the medieval period, clergy struggled to differentiate between "organic madness" and "divine rapture" (Mazzoni, 1996, p. 10). To be sure, the relationship was a fraught one in a religious context that had historically taken pride in "the madness of the cross." As Mazzoni notes about early Christianity, "Many of its most basic teachings (the belief in the resurrection of the dead, for example) seemed sheer madness to the classical mind. Early Christian, in their eagerness to differentiate their beliefs from hegemonic pagan philosophy, accepted and even celebrated this accusation of insanity and hence of dissenting difference." After all, she concludes, "his own mother and relatives took Christ for mad and threatened to tie him up, as the third chapter of the Gospel of Mark narrates" (Mazzoni, 1996, p. 10). Often the distinction between madness, demonic possession, and sanctity was unclear to casual observers. Even Angela of Foligno (1248–1309 CE), now canonized and widely recognized as one of the most significant mystics, was initially greeted as a madwoman by her townsmen after she gave away all of her belongings and began having rapturous visions in public.

Fraught as the distinction between madness and divine rapture was, authority figures did draw it and those authority figures were men. These men did more than simply diagnose, legitimize, or delegitimize female mystical experiences; they explicitly controlled the texts we have today recounting female mystical experiences, sometimes by demanding revisions when a first draft was too heterodox, sometimes by recording the words of illiterate women, and sometimes by writing hagiographies that reinterpreted their lives. As Hollywood (2002) argues, these editorial decisions were influenced by a range of factors that led the male clergy to emphasize the corporeal nature of female religious experience over women's internal experiences of their raptures.

Some of these influences were political. During the heyday of medieval mysticism, the Catholic Church was at war with the Cathars, a Christian sect that emphasized bodily renunciation and allowed women a relatively generous role within their communities. Stressing the bodily raptures, mortifications, and convulsions that would look so familiar to Charcot was partly a rhetorical move. It differentiated Catholic religiosity from the ascetic, body-denying beliefs of the Cathars, while simultaneously creating a new, acceptable model of religious expression for women within the Catholic Church (Hollywood, 2002, p. 254–55). Individual clergymen who wrote about these women or acted as their confessors were also incentivised to emphasize their raptures as a way of bolstering their own authority by borrowing the luster of their subjects. Jacques de Vitry (c. 1160/70–1240 CE), for example, re-counted in his *Life of Marie d'Oignies* that Marie made him her spiritual mouthpiece on her deathbed, charging him with the task of continuing her fight against heresy (Hollywood, 2002, p. 255).

Such political and personal motivations sometimes led men to exaggerate the somatic symptoms of raptures at the expense of the internal experiences described by female mystics. Hollywood (2002) gives as an example the story of Beatrice of Nazareth (c. 1200-1268 CE), who was a member of a women's religious movement during the late Middle Ages. Shortly after she died, someone, likely the abbess of her convent, commissioned an account of her life. Much of the third book was drawn from Beatrice's one surviving treatise, "Seven Manners of Loving God." Through close textual analysis, Hollywood shows that her hagiographer systematically literalized Beatrice's metaphors in his account of her life, turning expressions of spiritual rapture into physical signs patterned after the bodily experiences of other medieval mystics. Thus, although Beatrice only described her soul overflowing, her hagiographer translates that experience into a bodily one, marked by tears and other corporeal signs (Hollywood, 2002, p. 248–50). Her body became the site of sanctification and proof of her connection to God, despite Bea-trice's own quiet insistence that her raptures had been experienced internally.

The physiological and religious history of thinking about women, hyster-ia, and spirituality creates problems and precedents for thinking about the doctors and patients alike at Salpêtrière. The tendency of medieval clergy-men to mold the accounts of mysticism to fit their needs calls into question the doctors' easy equation of nineteenth-century hysteria with mysticism. If some unknown number of hagiographies of women were written to conform to the demands of a genre, as in Beatrice's case, rather than to record what really happened, there is no way of knowing how closely the behavior of one woman venerated as a mystic and another diagnosed as a hysteric actually resembled each other. Someone like Geneviève, who was extremely pious, might be mimicking the symptoms of the hagiographies she had grown up reading, rather than independently manifesting the symptoms of an ahistori-cal illness that had persisted unchanged from the medieval period to present.

Medieval hagiographers also provide a precedent for thinking about Char-cot's interest in the visible signs of hysteria, rather than more internalized states, like psychosis. Any number of scholars have remarked on the role photography played in Charcot's analysis of hysteria. In a reappraisal of feminist interpretations of hysteria, Cecily Devereux argued that Charcot's photographs were a medical attempt to "fix" the symptoms of hysteria into a stable set of visible symptoms. "This fixing pertains to the static representa-tion of the figure in Charcot's museum—the woman 'caught' in a hysterical posture (which necessitated her actually holding the pose in order for the camera to 'catch' it)—and to the fixing that is the photographic process. It also pertains to the fixing that is the attempt to stabilize meaning" (Devereux, 2014, p. 30). Photography created the illusion of orderly, universal poses out of the confusion of thrashing hysterics. In a very real sense, it created the disorder as a set of knowable, predictable symptoms. Yet it also had the strange result of minimizing the content of her visions—which is to say, minimizing the details of the psychotic dimension to the hysterical diagnosis.

This emphasis on the visible, somatic signs of religious experience over the content of Geneviève's visions will have direct bearing on my question for the final section: did the medical interpretation of Geneviève's symptoms help or exacerbate her suffering?

SUFFERING AND SELF-INTERPRETATION

I began this piece by arguing that hysteria provides a unique opportunity to ask frankly whether medical interpretations of Geneviève's visions and symptoms did a superior job alleviating her suffering compared to religious interpretations. Asking that question of contemporary psychiatry is too fraught of a question to address with any level of objectivity but hysteria, I reasoned, was a largely defunct diagnostic category that could be approached with some level of disinterestedness. The first section of this chapter high-lighted the difficulty of using contemporary definitions of psychosis and religious experience, arguing instead Geneviève's symptoms were better understood though the terminology of "hysteria" current in her day. In doing so, I sketched the conflicts among the religious, scientific, and scholarly interpretative frameworks, each of which sought to single out certain relig-ious experiences as pathological in order to consolidate their own authority to define the "true" nature of religion. The second section argued that the hysteric provided a particularly fertile case study for these debates over the nature of religion because there was a long history of understanding women's bodies as uniquely biologically and spiritually vulnerable to disruptive forces. Charcot and the other doctors of Salpêtrière participated in that tradi-tion, both by emphasizing the visible, somatic manifestations of women's religious experiences and by casting themselves as male authority figures capable of interpreting opaque symptoms.

In this final section, I want to tie the last two sections together by return-ing to my initial question about the efficacy of early psychiatry for alleviat-ing suffering. In this section, Geneviève takes her place as one of a long line of women who struggled with male authority figures over the right to inter-pret her symptoms. While biographical details suggest that Geneviève saw her identification with Louise Lateau as a form of escape from the suffering caused by a medical establishment that labeled her a hysteric, I will argue

Charcot's model of religion qua hysteria provided the only validation available of Geneviève's understanding of herself as touched by God.

On the surface, the question of whether the medical establishment made Geneviève's suffering better or worse seems trivial. Countless biographical details in Geneviève's life attest to her hostility toward the doctors at Salpêtrière. At times she threatened doctors, once chasing Charcot himself out of her room with the shout "Just wait until I get my hands on you!" (Hustvedt, 2001, p. 247). She escaped from various hospitals, including Salpêtrière, with some regularity (Hustvedt, 2011, p. 233–35). She once attempted suicide by hoarding her belladonna pills until she had a lethal dose, then swallowing them all. During hysterical episodes, her doctors recorded her reflecting on her life saying, "Poor Geneviève! . . . Your existence is so sad" (cited in Hustvedt, 2011, p. 252). Her entire pilgrimage to Lateau—itself following an escape from the hospital—attest to a profound desire on her part to break from a medical system that offered her little respect and autonomy by rewriting her life as one of a woman touched by God. None of these actions suggest a woman contented or grateful or even resigned to her role as a patient within an asylum. They all suggest a deep desire on Geneviève's part to reinterpret her life.

There are several different ways of thinking about why she turned toward a religious interpretation of her symptoms as most empowering. The first comes from the perspective of religious studies through the suggestion made by the famed anthropologist Clifford Geertz about why religion is peculiarly good at alleviating suffering. In his seminal work, *The Interpretation of Cultures,* he recounts the story of an old Ila woman. As the story progresses, she is slowly stripped of first her husband, then her children, then her grandchildren, until she is left totally alone. Desolate, she sets out on a search for her god, "Leza, the Besetting One," to ask why she has suffered such loss. She goes from country to country, looking for the end of the earth where she might find a road to God. In each country, the natives would ask her why she came. She would answer by telling her story and ask if they had ever met anyone who had suffered like she did. And in each country the response she got was the same. "Yes, we see! That is how you are! Bereaved of friends and husband? In what do you differ from others? The Besetting One sits on all of our backs and we cannot shake him off" (Geertz, 1973, p. 104). The old woman never finds God and so the story ends as she dies of heartbreak.

Geertz is too sophisticated a thinker to imagine religion exists to deny or paper over the existence of suffering. If anything, he points out, religion often actively glorifies suffering—One only has to think of any of the Christian iconography of the crucified Christ to grasp his point. He argues that one of the main roles of religion is to make "suffering sufferable" by formulating a worldview through symbols that gives order to what William James once called "the blooming, buzzing confusion" of life. "The effort," Geertz insists, "is not to deny the undeniable—that there are unexplained events, that life hurts, or that rain falls on the just—but to deny that there are inexplicable events, that life is unendurable, and that justice is a mirage" (Geertz, 1973, p. 108). We can presume that Geneviève's pilgrimage offered her the chance to make her suffering sufferable by giving it order and meaning. Without a religious framework, she was a disintegrating personality, prone to fits of rage, lust, hallucinations, and self-mutilation. Within a religious framework, she was a pious woman whose tenuous grasp on reality was not a tragedy, but a sign of God's grace. Under Geertz's reading, then, Geneviève turned toward a religious interpretation of her suffering because religion is uniquely suited to narrativizing suffering in such a way as to make it bearable.

Geertz has been accused of providing an ahistorical, universalizing account of religion, however (Asad, 1993). A slightly different account of why Geneviève sought to reinterpret her life through a religious lens comes from Eric J. Cassell's classic work, *The Nature of Suffering and the Goals of Medicine*. For Cassell, himself a doctor writing for other doctors, it is important not to confuse pain with suffering. Pain, he thinks, can be a source of suffering, particularly if it is severe enough, its cause is unknown, its duration seems limitless, or if it signals a catastrophic condition (Cassell, 2004, p. 35). For Cassell, culture played a key role in determining what an individual might experience as suffering. At its most basic, suffering occurs when a patient's sense of herself as a whole, intact person is threatened. A person, for Cassell, consists of an individual's personality, past life experiences, family, cultural background, politics, habits, body, secret life, perceived future, and spiritual life. Suffering happens when events damage the webs of relationships that make up a person, whether by threatening death or creating the more nebulous fear that an experience will overwhelm or transform a person so totally that she will become unrecognizable to herself (Cassell, 2004, p. 42). The logical extension of this definition of suffering is that something that would seem catastrophic in one context might not register as suffering at all, if social bonds can accommodate an experience without receiving damage. This logic leads Cassell to draw back from labelling the deprivations of saints and ascetics suffering. If "great pain or deprivation" leads a person to feel she has become closer to God, she might not feel as if she has suffered at all. She might, instead, feel a sense of triumph (Cassell, 2004, p. 34). In this reading, religion would allow Geneviève to reframe her ecstasies as reinforcing her place in society, rather than threatening her sense of self.

Alternately, a third way of understanding the solace religion gave Geneviève might be found by turning to feminist interpretations of hysteria. In the wake of Freud and psychoanalysis more generally, a number of female scholars begin reimagining hysteria as a form of protest against patriarchal oppression. French feminists, most famously Luce Irigaray and Helène Cixous, argued that psychoanalysis enshrined male psychology and physiology as the norm. By contrast, women were defined negatively, or as secondary subjects who lacked and envied the phallus (Devereux, 2014, p. 25). Hysteria in particular, due to the long history of attributing it to a malfunction of the womb, was a diagnosis that reinforced the nineteenth century equation of women with their biological capacity to bear children.

Accordingly, for many twentieth-century feminists, early hysterics like Geneviève were not ill. Rather, they translated their distress at the constraints and expectations of sexist society into symptoms, creating in the process, as Showalter phrased it, "a specifically feminine protolanguage, communicating through the body messages that cannot be verbalized" (Showalter, 1993, p. 286). Some critics, like Showalter, have questioned the efficacy of hysteria as a form of social protest, arguing that by accepting the idea that hysteria is a female disease feminists have reduced women to their biology and erased the existence of male hysterics (Showalter, 1993). Nevertheless, this feminist reading of hysteria offers a third way of understanding why Geneviève sought a religious understanding of her symptoms. It was a doubled form of protest. Both her symptoms and her rejection of the label of hysteria could be seen as rebellion against a society that had consigned her to early child labor, denied her any stable family life, labelled her genetically degenerate, took her child from her, and subjected her to medical treatments that were often brutal and humiliating.

I am sympathetic to all of these interpretations in varying degrees. I think, however, that reading Geneviève's pilgrimage to Louise Lateau as a straight-forward rejection of the medical interpretation of her symptoms in order to alleviate her pain is too simplistic. That narrative falls once again into the trap of painting the relationship between religion and medicine as starkly oppositional during this time.

As I noted earlier when I quoted the Belgian physician who examined Louise Lateau, the Catholic Church had a vested interested in labelling some women as sick rather than saintly. Their willingness to concede that some number of women suffered nervous disorders, despite the apparently religious nature of their behavior, gave a certain level of respectability and credence to those cases they did authenticate. It also allowed the Church to position itself as an institution concerned with all truth, not merely theological. No longer was the Church the same institution that had condemned Galileo, this rhetoric suggested. It was scientific, modern, and just as skeptical of false claims to sanctity as the most positivistic physician.

What this meant concretely for Geneviève was that the Church was highly unlikely to validate her interpretations of her visions. This claim is not mere speculation. Geneviève had spent time in the care of Catholic nuns and they had responded with distinct skepticism toward her. After her first hysterical attack at the age of sixteen, Geneviève had further contact with nuns when she was sent to a hospital staffed, like most hospitals of the time, by nuns. As part of her condition, Geneviève began displaying the signs of a hysterical pregnancy. Her abdomen swelled, she ate erratically, and vomited frequently. During her daily attacks, when she would convulse and throw her head against the wall, the nuns berated her for trying to murder her child. In one doctor's words, they "persecuted" (Hustvedt, 2011, p. 231) Geneviève, and when, in time, they discovered she was not pregnant, they transferred her to the lunatic asylum.

Part of their response was likely due to the beliefs circulating at the time that degeneracy was a hereditary trait. As presumably the abandoned child of an unwed mother, the wisdom of the day held that Geneviève was likely to become an unwed mother in turn. Her swollen abdomen validated those preconceptions. As she aged and became pregnant in truth, those conceptions would have been confirmed. Part of the skepticism of the Church likely would have been caused by the content of her visions, however.

As I noted at the start of the first section, Geneviève's visions had at least two main themes. The first was religious. She fell into raptures, had visions of God, and believed herself to be in the presence of the sacred. The second theme was erotic. It is genuinely difficult to parse how much of her erotic history was hallucinated. It could very well be that Camille had been a real, deceased lover, rather than a hallucination. Likewise, it is also within the realm of possibility that she was having an affair with a doctor. She had done so once before; she escaped one of the early hospitals she was committed to by running away with a medical intern (Hustvedt, 2011, p. 233). Regardless of the veracity of these particular stories, her hospital records clearly record that she could switch abruptly from an ecstatic religious vision to an explicitly sexual one. As one doctor wrote, "Geneviève would fall back on her bed, lift her chemise and spread her thighs; or she would address one of her attendants, abruptly leaning toward him and saying, 'Kiss me! . . . Give me! . . . Here, here's my . . . ' And her gestures further accentuate the meaning of her words" (cited in Hustvedt, 2011, p. 257). Another doctor, Paul Richer, wrote on that subject that, "Most often her hallucinations are lecherous. She sees Camille, calls out to him: 'Camille, I have never loved anyone but you.' She affects theatrical poses accompanied by these words: 'Give me your love. Don't insult me.' Or else she assumes silent poses, approaching ecstasy" (Hustvedt, 2011, p. 257).

Much has been made of the erotic language of medieval mystics, who often described themselves as "brides of Christ" and recounted erotically charged visions. By the early twentieth century, the practice of retroactively diagnosing figures like Teresa of Ávila as hysterics and sublimated erotomaniac had become relatively commonplace (Mazzoni, 1996, p. 46). At risk of stating the obvious, though, there is a wide and nontrivial gap from the perspective of religious authority between using erotically charged language in describing visions of God and imploring bystanders to have sex. From a psychoanalytic account, like that of Jacques Lacan, the content of visions might matter less than the libidinal forces driving them (see Mazzoni 1996, p. 46). But from the perspective of an institution that had spent centuries carefully monitoring women's visions, the slide from metaphorical ecstasy to call for literal, carnal love is the difference between orthodoxy and heterodoxy.

Without a doubt, blithely equating female mystics to hysterics is a sexist move that, in Mazzoni's succinct formulation proceeds, "from an ideology that is not pressed to take into serious account the mystic's accomplishments and her texts" (Mazzoni, 2006, p. 4). In Geneviève's case, however, the willingness of her doctors to collapse her explicitly sexual visions into the eroticized language of medieval saints was more than merely sexist. Rather, I contend Bourneville, Charcot, and Geneviève's other doctors were able to ignore or rationalize the mixed content of Geneviève's visions because they systematically minimized the psychotic dimension of hysteria in favor of its outward manifestations.

Charcot had always emphasized visible signs of hysteria over the account of his patients about their mental states. That was why he focused so much on photography and looked to old paintings, rather than texts, for signs that hysteria had existed in the past. In a certain respect, it was only natural that his belief that hysteria could be recognized by external signs alone would lead him to privilege inordinately the parallels between religious and hysterical behavior. Thus, for Bourneville, proof of Geneviève's hysteria could be found in her nipple amputation, which marked her an ascetic like the Russian sect of the Skoptzy (Hustvedt, 2011, p. 238) and her extreme fasting, which hearkened back to Catherine of Siena. Likewise, for Charcot, the details of her grimaces could be compared with paintings of demoniacs and photographs to create diagnostic tools for hysteria. Hysteria and religion alike were recognized by their visible manifestations.

As I noted, this bias toward somatic signs of altered states of consciousness was hardly unique to Charcot. Medieval hagiographers had translated women's mystical experiences into bodily signs of God's presence, as noted earlier, but they did so in their capacity as editors, censors, and translators of women's religious experiences. The difference was that Charcot focused on the external at the expense of the content of visions. The Church has always cared about the content of visions, in addition to bodily signs of it.

Counterintuitively, however, this emphasis on external signs of religiosity provided an opportunity for Geneviève. The Church might not have been willing to sanctify her, given her mixed, lustful hallucinations of Camille, but her doctors were perfectly happy to discard or explain away the heterodox nature of her visions. She may have been sick, according to the medical regime, but her religious visions were affirmed as real in a perverse way—

real, at least, as any other religious vision. The only problem is that, according to that same regime, her religious ecstasies were pathological and had no value.

That, I think, is the tragedy of Geneviève's life and also what makes it so difficult in the final analysis to separate the religious and medical interpretations of her life. Religion offered a way out for Geneviève. It offered a form of rebellion, escape, and the possibility of a radical reinterpretation of her life as closer to the venerated Belgian ascetic, rather than the madwomen in the lunatic ward. And yet sanctity does not take place in a void, as noted by Marzanski and Bratton (Marzanski and Bratton, 2002, p. 361). It requires social sanctification by some sort of external body; otherwise, it is perceived as mere, self-involved delusion. For all that the medical establishment distressed her and used her case history for its own purposes, it gave her that validation.

CONCLUSION

The question of whether Geneviève was religious or ill, or religious *and* ill, is, in the final analysis, less a question about how to understand her life than one of how to understand religion I have argued that Charcot and his colleagues at Salpêtrière developed diagnostic criteria that focused on external signs of hysteria over the hysteric's account of her state. The belief that religious ecstasy was a form of hysteria led, naturally enough, to the minimization of any difference in the internal experiences of hysterics and mystics that might trouble the equation of the two. In this minimization of internal experiences, psychosis played a liminal but important role. The critical force of calling mystics hysterics depended on the implicit belief that visions were psychotic—that is, untethered from reality and rooted in some sort of pathological condition yet to be discovered. Yet too much attention to the content of such "psychotic" visions might have forced Geneviève's doctors to start asking more pointed questions about the etiology of different categories of visions and whether Geneviève's mixture of sexual and pious visions really could be mapped seamlessly on to the raptures of saints. In short, their equation of religion and hysteria drew primarily on external similarities in behavior but relied implicitly on the normative force of declaring all visions some form of hallucinatory loss of contact with reality.

Without a doubt, the attitude toward religion displayed in Salpêtrière was reductive. Beneath the belief that hysteria could be diagnosed through paintings, though, some interesting, subtle questions were buried. Is religion best recognized by what people feel and write, or what they do? How can you differentiate between the psychotic and spiritual? When should you privilege a first-person account of a spiritual experience, particularly when it violates pre-existing scientific beliefs?

As for Charcot, in his later years he began to feel doubt about the years he had spent insisting that hysteria was a neurological disease. In 1892, toward the end of his life, he wrote a small essay on faith healing that suggested hysteria might be a psychological disease that could be cured by the power of suggestion. He died a year later, so we can never know if the piece represented a softening of his attitude toward medieval mystics or toward the social utility of religion more broadly. Nor, for that matter, do we know what Geneviève would have made of this concession by her old doctor. The last record of her is from 1878. It recounts a fight with Charcot. A short time after, she left Salpêtrière, disappearing from the clinic and the records.

REFERENCES

Adair, M. (1996). Plato's View of the 'Wandering Uterus.' *The Classical Journal*, 91(2), 153–63.

American Psychiatric Association. (2013). Schizophrenia Spectrum and Other Psychotic Disorders. In *Diagnostic and statistical manual of mental disorders* (5th ed.). Washington, DC: Author. https://doi.org/10.1176/appi.books.9780890425596.dsm02.

Asad, T. (1993). *Genealogies of religion: discipline and reasons of power in Christianity and Islam*. Baltimore: Johns Hopkins University Press.

Batnitzky, L. F. (2011). *How Judaism became a religion: An introduction to modern Jewish thought*. Princeton, NJ: Princeton University Press.

Brett, C. (2002). Spiritual experience and psychopathology: Dichotomy or interaction? *Philosophy, Psychiatry, & Psychology*, 9(4), 373–80. doi:10.1353/ppp.2003.0055.

Bourneville, D. M. (1878). Science et miracle. *Louise Lateau, ou la stigmatisée belge*. Paris: V.A. Delahaye.

Bynum, C. W. (1987). *Holy feast and holy fast: The religious significance of food to medieval women*. Berkeley: University of California Press.

Cassell, E. J. (2004). *The nature of suffering and the goals of medicine*. New York: Oxford University Press.

Chidester, D. (1996). *Savage systems: colonialism and comparative religion in southern Africa*. Charlottesville: University Press of Virginia.

Devereux, C. (2014). *Hysteria, feminism, and gender revisited: The case of the second wave*. ESC: English Studies in Canada, 40(1), 19–45. doi:10.1353/esc.2014.0004.

Diagnostic and statistical manual of mental disorders: DSM-5. (2013). Washington, D.C.: American Psychiatric Association.

Didi-Huberman, G., & Charcot, J. M. (2003). *Invention of hysteria: Charcot and the photographic iconography of the Salpêtrière*. Cambridge, MA: MIT Press.

Fulford, K. W., & Jackson, M. (1997). Spiritual experience and psychopathology. *Philosophy, Psychiatry, & Psychology*, 4(1), 41–65. doi:10.1353/ppp.1997.0002.

Geertz, C. (1973). *The interpretation of cultures: Selected essays*. New York: Basic Books.

Goetz, C. G., Bonduelle, M., & Gelfand, T. (1995). *Charcot: Constructing neurology*. New York: Oxford University Press.

Hollywood, A. M. (2002). *Sensible ecstasy: Mysticism, sexual difference, and the demands of history*. Chicago: University of Chicago Press.

Hustvedt, A. (2011). *Medical muses: Hysteria in nineteenth-century Paris*. New York: W.W. Norton & Co.

Kugelmann, R. (2011). *Psychology and Catholicism: Contested boundaries*. Cambridge: Cambridge University Press.

Lefebvre, F. J., & Northcote, J. S. (1873). *Louise Lateau of Bois d'Haine: Her life, her ecstasies, and her stigmata, a medical study.* London: Burnes and Oates.

Marzanski, M., & Bratton, M. (2002). Psychopathological symptoms and religious experience: A critique of Jackson and Fulford. *Philosophy, Psychiatry, & Psychology*, 9(4), 359–71. doi:10.1353/ppp.2003.0062.

Masuzawa, T. (2005). *The invention of world religions, or, How European universalism was preserved in the language of pluralism.* Chicago: University of Chicago Press.

Mazzoni, C. (1996). *Saint hysteria: Neurosis, mysticism, and gender in European culture.* Ithaca, NY: Cornell University Press.

Nongbri, B. (2013). *Before religion: a history of a modern concept.* New Haven: Yale University Press.

Scull, A. (2009). *Hysteria: The biography.* Oxford: Oxford University Press.

Schizophrenia Spectrum and Other Psychotic Disorders. (n.d.). Retrieved January 08, 2017, from http://dsm.psychiatryonline.org/doi/abs/10.1176/appi.books.9780890425596.dsm.02.

Showalter, E. (1993). Hysteria, feminism, and gender hysteria. In S. Gilman. *Hysteria beyond Freud.* (286–344). Berkeley: University of California Press.

Spinoza, B. D., & Morgan, M. L. (2006). *The essential Spinoza: Ethics and related writings.* Indianapolis: Hackett Pub.

Psychosis. (n.d.) In Oxford English dictionary online. (n.d.). Oxford: Oxford University Press. Retrieved from https://en.oxforddictionaries.com/definition/psychosis.

Chapter Seven

From Sick to Gifted

Discovering Shamanic Illness

Gogo Ekhaya Esima

I was the first born of a single mother in a small Midwestern town populated mostly by white people. My sisters and I had humble beginnings. Our days were spent playing in the back yard, on project playgrounds, and neighborhood railroad tracks. We looked forward to the day our mother would receive her monthly check, which was just enough to pay the rent and bills. On lucky occasions we would be treated to a trip to Kmart to get a new dress, hair barrette, or anything that made us feel like pretty little girls. I was always a quiet, little, shy girl, especially around adults. I was the dreamy child, inspecting the sunflowers, creating art and new dance moves to entertain the family at backyard barbecues and birthday parties. I spent days with extended family, aunts, uncles, cousins, and the like. In my African American community, family was always our place of comfort where we could just let loose and be who we were.

I don't remember a time when I didn't know my father. He was around a lot during my early years, I'd see him at least every week. My mom would always say, "You know I could never be with your father but we are the best of friends." My dad was this big, 6'1" creative giant. He was a poet, a chef, a teacher, and an amazing artist. I was always inspired by his vast knowledge and it seemed like he knew a little about everything. But, the boundaries of our relationship were very thin and confusing for me as a child. Sleepovers at his home were fun and eventful. We would watch National Geographic and cooking shows on TV, take long walks visiting friends and family, and his comedian-like personality would always have me laughing belly up. I looked forward to the meals he prepared, with dishes from all over the world. I liked this man during the day, but at night the alcohol took precedence, and this is where the line between father and daughter became very blurry for me. He would always have me close at night and I don't remember a time when the touching and molestation wasn't present. Eventually, I told my mother and she did her best to help me and decided to press charges. I remember being in the detective's office with little dolls and private parts to demonstrate what had happened behind closed doors with my father. When my dad was put away in a detention center for a few months, I was told that it was because he had a warrant for his arrest and had stolen something. After his release, my mom decided that it was okay for me to see my dad again. At his request, I was dropped off at a local playground to meet him. The entire time he told me how wrong I was about the molestation and that I had over-exaggerated and lied. He asked if it would be okay if we tried again to be daughter and dad. So, from as early as I could remember, I was always confused and distrustful of relationships and adults. That confusion created deep anxiety throughout my years growing up but I continued to move through life as if nothing had happened, because that is how I was taught to present myself in front of others. "It's all over, forget about it." My mother would say "Don't no one else need to know our family business, you hear." I remember one night my dad was at a friend's party, drinking in the basement, and called me downstairs. He stared intensely into my eyes and told me that he was going to die soon, and that I should be strong and continue to be a good student so I could be successful in life, better than him. I remember being extremely scared because I instinctively knew that he was talking about suicide.

I was molested by other men that were in my family and in close relation to it. I truly believed that there was something about me that made these people feel it was ok to touch me. As I grew older, my father became addicted to crack; eventually my mother as well, after being involved in several unhealthy marriages and relationships. I was in high school at the time, and dropped out for a while to work more hours at my job, since my mother was out in the streets and never home. I was heartbroken—I never thought my mom would be the one to use drugs, she barely ever drank alcohol and was always against drug use. During this time, I had begun attending church at one of my best friends' parishes and felt such a strong connection there. It was the place where the weight I was carrying could be forgotten, my source of release at the time. This is where spirituality started to play an important role in my life. I had committed myself wholeheartedly to building a relationship with God and it changed my life completely. I was involved in every aspect of the church setting: choir practice, Wednesday night prayer service, Bible study, youth group and Sunday services, both morning and night. Something about being exposed to a supportive community drew me in, offering me a family setting complete with positive male role models, brother and sisterhood, inspirational women, grandmothers, and children who reminded me of cousins.

During this time, I was also connected to spirit in a way I had never experienced before. My heart opened, I could be vulnerable and cry when I needed to, and dance and shout for joy. I felt a sense of connection and belonging. One day while in church praying, I heard a voice say "You have a calling." At that time, I interpreted this calling to mean as an evangelist or minister. I was filled with excitement and immediately told my pastor of the news. He looked at me like a father would when his daughter came in from outdoors playing and exclaiming that she was going to build a spaceship to travel to another galaxy when she grew up. I received a pat on the shoulder, "You're young, let's see what happens," he said. I expected him to swoop me up and start teaching me how to answer my calling. Instead, I left his office with disappointment and feeling that he didn't fully believe what this holy voice had told me.

After years of committing to a holy way of life in this church, it all came crashing down after being sexually assaulted by a fellow parishioner whom I had trusted. I confided with a few women from the church about what had happened, and was scorned for being around a married man "in all my youthfulness." This was all too familiar and the circle of distrust, blame, and abuse was standing in front of me once again. I broke all ties to the church community; the place I once believed was sacred. I also turned my back on my spiritual calling.

I went through life, got married, and started a family. However, it became harder and harder for me to deal with the pain that I was carrying inside. When I was intimate with my husband, I would see my father's face and push him off me in anger. Everything around me seemed to be falling apart. My relationship with my children became intense. I was afraid to breastfeed because my perspective on the intimacy and nurturing a parent has with their children had become distorted. I became angry and emotionally unstable. During two of my pregnancies I became severely depressed and suicidal. I had my first psychiatric hospitalization while pregnant. I separated from my husband while carrying our third child. Shortly after he was born we divorced.

The thought of ending my life never went away. When a challenge or hardship arose, it was the place that I went to, the solution to the chaos around and within me. I tried therapy a few times and gave up after the first visits because I never felt a connection or sensed that the therapist understood my experiences. I started to take psychiatric drugs for the first time outside of inpatient treatment and felt foggy and emotionally disconnected to everything around me, including my children. They would approach me with excitement or in a playful manner and I couldn't even respond with a smile. I decided that this medication was not worth the side effects, which took away my ability to experience the joy of my children. I began realizing that I needed to connect to my creative energy again and find something that could bring back my passion for life. I started writing poems. Coming from a family full of artists and poets, this gift came naturally. The writing fueled something deep inside me. Eventually I started performing with groups of friends and fellow artists. I had found community again—I felt alive.

The traumas I had experienced wanted to surface through my writing and eventually I allowed them to. I shared poems about my experiences and people in the audience would be deeply moved by my passion to tell my story. Each time I stepped onto stage, it was a healing release for me, but throughout this artistic calling, I was still experiencing a wave of emotions that I couldn't handle. I noticed that the mother I had always dreamed of being for my children was the opposite of what I truly was. I did not want my children to experience my sickness, my anger. I decided to run away to another city, promising that I'd be back for them in a year's time. I just needed a break, time to find out who I was and cultivate my artistic goals.

About eight months after moving, I found out that my father had died and the family had chosen me to coordinate his funeral. I flew back home and did what I had to do, although it took every ounce of courage I had left to do it. I spoke a few words at my father's funeral from an inspirational book that I had recently read. I spoke aloud about the need for unity in our family but inside I was a raging child wanting to let all the dust out from underneath the rug and tell the sobbing audience what this evil man had done to his daughter. When I returned home, I felt beaten up. Again, I had to wear the mask of the strong woman. The little dark place inside of me where I carried all my wounds had grown into something massive.

It came to the point that I wasn't able to handle the artistic energy that I had been channeling. I was feeling more overwhelmed than inspired by it. I became more sensitive as time went on and began to feel anxious about going on stage and sharing my work. By then I had joined a band and my friends could see the change in me. I would want to be in the background and would feel nauseous at the thought of standing in front of a microphone. My entire body would tremor. Eventually I decided to leave the band. My friends were terribly disappointed that I had dismantled our dream to make music for a living, which in turn made me climb even deeper within my sinking hole. I began self-medicating with marijuana and food. I would wake up in the morning and smoke until it was time to sleep again. Empty pints of ice cream and containers of cookies littered my bed. I began reaching out to men whom I'd thought would be a comfort to my depression. I would barely call them relationships because it was simply a detrimental exchange of energy, sex, food, and drugs. I had lost stable housing and ended up rooming with a guy I was seeing. I began drinking alcohol on a daily basis at this point. It was the only way that I could be romantically available to my partner. I taught him how to use me, and my lifelessness opened up the doors of abuse on many levels. Suicide was still a constant in my thoughts. I could not sustain employment. With all of my talents and skill, I would land a great opportunity and my emotional and spiritual instability would destroy everything.

I was juggling three jobs at one time when the visions and voices started to creep in. I was living with my guy friend in a tiny room. I had gotten used to locking myself in this room; I did not trust the old man we were renting from who also shared the apartment. I became very suspicious. I was afraid to walk down the hallway to use the restroom or even shower. I was sitting in my bed one night and, as clear as day, my deceased father was standing four feet away from me. He continued to appear from that night forward and it was scaring the shit out of me. The veil of social reality was dissolving. I could sense other people's emotions so vividly, that I would just hide in my room. I wanted to drown the visions and voices that were haunting me.

The voices would tell me to cut myself, to go walk into traffic, and to take bottles of pills. I listened. I no longer wanted to be here in this world, the place where nothing seemed to fit, especially me. I spent many weeks in locked psychiatric units after my suicide attempts. One particular hospital offered art therapy and tai chi classes, and had a visiting monk who led meditation groups. Throughout the fog of all the heavily sedating psychotropic drugs and sleeping pills, I was able to connect to something within these groups, connect to something familiar within myself. But, the medications did not stop my haunting visions or the urges to harm myself.

While sitting in meditation, I had a pleasant vision of a scarab beetle and a wolf. In art therapy, I painted what I had witnessed and later did some research as to what these animals might mean from a spiritual perspective. I felt that what I was experiencing was somehow spiritually connected but I was not sure how or why. The beetle had a message, beetles symbolize the ability to survive, transform, and experience rebirth. The wolf's message was balance, harmony, inner knowing, and new beginnings. These messages resonated with my spirit and in them I found inspiration. I was released from the hospital and placed into a homeless shelter.

The hostile environment of New York City homeless shelters completely rocked my emotional stability. I ended up back in the psych ward, only this time I was threatened to be placed in a long-term locked facility or state hospital. So, for me it felt like a choice between state hospital, being homeless, or going back to the abusive relationship that I had left back in the tiny room. I chose the tiny room. I had a load of medication to help me sleep through the chaos and battles of my voices and visions.

Upon my discharge it was mandatory that I attend a partial hospitalization program. I was lucky, because, unlike many day treatment programs for recipients of mental health services, this one also included art therapy and meditation. This part of treatment motivated me enough to get out of bed every morning and go to the program. After I graduated, I was referred to a Dialectical Behavioral Therapy program, which I despised. Group therapy was very intense for me as my ultra-sensitivities would expand with each person's story and wounds.

At home in the tiny room, I was still being abused and still under the influence of drugs; the street drugs had simply changed to prescribed medications. Somehow the message of the wolf and beetle was still pushing me through, I could almost taste the transformation to come. I found out about a program that was run by people called "Peers," meaning individuals with lived experience of mental health challenges. They offered music, studio recording, art, peer support groups, and guitar lessons. It seemed right up my alley so I checked them out. Here is where I met people who were like me and were doing amazing things. It was the first time I heard the word "recovery." This word did not fly around in the psychiatrists' offices, therapeutic sessions, or hospitals that I had been to. The peer experience was all about "I see myself in you" and "this is my recovery journey, let me hear yours." I was in total awe. For the first time, I felt and witnessed a sense of hope after my diagnosis. I learned that I did not have to become or even identify with my diagnosis, that it was ok, it did not have to be the center of my life. Here I found a family again and this time one that did not seek to change who I was, change my experiences, or cover them up. I could be who I was with all my flaws, and be accepted and appreciated.

I ended up becoming a Peer specialist and began training to counsel individuals, run support groups, and share my gifts. The organization that I worked for was staffed with over 90 percent peers including the CEO. What an inspiration, what a beautiful movement to be part of. I learned about the history of the Peer movement and how many people fought to have their voices heard, especially fierce women like Sally Zinman, Judi Chamberlin, Mary Ellen Copeland, and Pat Deegan, who have been fighting for a very long time for positive change in our mental health system. I now had a work environment that supported my personal wellness and recovery, and the opportunity to be of service to those with shared experiences. My transformation was beginning. After working part-time for a few months, I was offered a full-time position that allowed me to get my own place and end the abusive relationship for good. Due to a conflicting work schedule, I could no longer continue the Dialectical Behavior Therapy program. I was told that I'd be referred to a different hospital's program for psychiatric care. This referral never happened, the ball was dropped somewhere. I attempted to set up care for myself, but every program I found either did not accept my insurance or had a waiting list of six weeks or more. When I inquired as to what to do about my prescription refills during the wait, I was informed that the quickest way was to go into the hospital's emergency room. I was petrified at the thought of having to go back to the hospital—the eerie familiarity of the cycles of trauma in psychiatric emergency rooms left an unforgettable stench under my nose. After finally experiencing what recovery could feel like, I could not go back. I decided to stop the medications.

I learned quickly that the decision to quit psychiatric medications cold turkey was just the same as quitting any street drug or alcohol addiction. I went through three months of hellish withdrawal, with night sweats, tremors, trouble sleeping, mood swings, and pain coursing through my joints and limbs. There were times when I could barely walk, yet still I was determined to show up for work; and when I couldn't I was supported by my co-workers, my fellow peers. The difference with this job was that I could openly share with them what I was doing and why I was doing it, because personal wellness was at the very forefront of our work. During this time, my job selected me and one other co-worker to attend a recovery program whose focus was using the foundations of Eastern healing, such as pranayama breathing, to facilitate self-healing in mental health. With this opportunity, and the reinforcement of my duty to maintain recovery, I made it through all the challenges and successfully withdrew from ten different medications. From that point on, I have always recommended to those who want to get off psychiatric medications to use harm reduction tools and work with a doctor, as I could have experienced even more dangerous symptoms than I did.

During my new-found recovery I began reconnecting to my spiritual self. I was seeking answers as to why I could see, feel, hear, and experience things that others didn't. I knew there was a deeper meaning than just symptoms of psychosis. I ended up spending nights researching spirituality and discovered traditional healing practices of indigenous communities and shamanism. I came across a book by Malidoma Patrice Somé entitled *Of Water and the Spirit*. The story about Somé's African shamanic initiation drew me in and a passion seated deep within my soul began to emerge. It was the inner knowing of the wolf whispering in my ears, activating a memory that I had forgotten. I could relate to Somé's experiences of realms outside of this concrete world. But in his story he wasn't ostracized, labeled, or mistreated because of it. Instead, he was held by a community that understood and supported him. I now had a deep desire to know who I was and why I was living. During my years of mental distress, this question would arise and there would be no answer that made sense. Yes, I knew that on some level I was here on this earth to bear children and be a mother, but what was a mother who did not have her children? My year away from them had turned into many years at this point in my life and left an even deeper wound within my spirit. I had recognized this wound and wanted more than anything to heal and make my way back to them.

While searching further into African Spirituality, I found a woman who was a Sangoma and a priestess in the Yoruba and Akan spiritual traditions. Sangoma are shamans or medicine people of South Africa. This woman was living in the United States, so I decided to book an appointment with her. We were on an online video conference and she gave me an Ancestral Divination, which is an ancient form of oracle reading practiced by many tribal cultures. Without knowing anything but my name, she told me a story about my life, my deepest secrets, my worries, my struggles, and my calling. She explained to me that in her tradition, the reason for my sickness was due to my life's purpose as a healer. Some call it a "shamanic illness," a symptom of the calling. Completing an initiation as a shaman would align me with my divine purpose, thus curing my illness. I was told that I had ancestor's way back in my lineage who were Sangoma and that they were passing their healing gifts to me through my DNA. I let a bellowing cry of release pour out from depths untapped—I knew that everything she'd said made complete and utter sense. I had finally found my answer. This woman, Yeye Gogo Nana, became my teacher.

I found that she had experiences very similar to mine and had gone through a spiritual emergence. She helped to me to further understand that I wasn't "crazy," and that my experience with seeing visions, hearing voices, and feeling deeply wasn't a disease but a gift. Through my initiation, I was able to explore these experiences while being held and supported by a community of women. I trained with other sisters who had the calling. I now had another strong family who did not judge me and held space for my experiences.

Exploring the spiritual realm is not an easy task and I've learned that one must be guided and not do it alone. When visual and auditory interruptions happen without a supportive community, it causes huge problems. We can see this every day, for instance, when arriving at a stoplight and noticing the lady on the corner, pushing a cart full of everything she owns, and talking out loud to no one that we can see. My journey opened up a whirlwind of inner demons that I had to face and learn how to fight for the first time in my life. But behind me were many Ancestral guardians to support me. I transitioned from being a battered ragdoll, running away in fear, into a weapon-carrying warrior spirit. I delved into the realm of the divine feminine and began the process of healing my sacred womb from accumulated traumas. I've had to meet each traumatic experience face-to-face with space for grieving, forgiveness, acceptance, and gratitude. I was not reliving it, but reviewing it, in the spiritual realm; meeting the experience from a new perspective with an understanding and knowing that only spirit could show me. Without the support of my divine ancestors, my teacher, and my spiritual sisters, I would continue to be haunted by this gift or maybe even be dead.

A beautiful gift it is. I learned how to cultivate my abilities to help myself and others heal. The haunting voices I experienced turned into voices that are helpful and now assist others. My visions went from toxic, to showing me the stories of other people's lives and ancestors. These transformations have become beautiful signs in my journey. I went through shamanic initiation while still being employed as a Peer. I was blessed to work with people who listened and accepted my spiritual journey.

It was difficult going through an African initiation in a Western society. I had to unlearn a lot of the ideas and teachings of the Western mindframe in order to be able receive what spirit had for me. Sangoma must undergo the harsh and stimulating initiation process to receive a title of healer. Sangoma are expert voices hearers and seers—we must use our gifts to find hidden or missing items and go through many other challenging tasks in order to complete training. With all of the overstimulation in our societies, it is challenging to go back to the ancient ways of our ancestors. As a result, many people begin the process of initiation but don't finish. Shamanic initiation is truly a lifelong process and commitment.

In South Africa, I discovered how important community really is when one experiences depression, emotional instability, hearing voices, or seeing visions. I have learned that it is much more beneficial to allow an individual space to sit with their experience and not try to drown them out, because space is where they can discover the learning and deep healing that wants to emerge. I've learned that a mental health system that ostracizes individuals and forces them into a particular mold is a failing one. Instead, people suffering from voices and vision should be accepted into a supportive community environment and given personalized tools to meet their own needs, truths, and recovery. I am grateful to be a woman, a healer, and mother who has reunited with her children and found her purpose in this lifetime—to be of service to a community that is begging for a major shift toward healing and empowerment.

IV

PSYCHIATRIC PERSPECTIVES ON WOMEN & PSYCHOSIS

Psychosis in Women

A Perspective from Psychiatry

Simone Ciufolini and Nicola Byrne

This chapter is written by two psychiatrists, both practicing clinically within the National Health Service in London, England. Simone Ciufolini has a background in academic psychiatry and continues as an active researcher in the field of psychosis within psychiatry. He is lead author for the sections below in the first part of this chapter, which provide some background definitions and outline the current scientific understanding of psychosis within the psychiatric literature. Nicola Byrne has worked as a consultant psychiatrist on an acute mental health unit for women in South London for over ten years. During this time, she has treated many hundreds of women presenting with what have been conceptualized as psychotic symptoms, in the broadest sense at least. The second part of this chapter sketches three fictionalized case studies drawn from her experience, describing common clinical challenges, dilemmas, and tensions that can arise in this context, especially when the perspectives of staff and patients can differ widely. This chapter is therefore an attempt to synthetize the academic literature with everyday experience. It is written solely from the perspective of psychiatric professionals and does not include the voice of women who have experienced psychosis themselves other than as filtered through our understanding—however incomplete that may be. We hope, therefore, this contribution will stand alongside in dialogue with the voices of women who have experienced psychosis featured elsewhere in this book.

DEFINITIONS & DISORDERS

How is the term psychosis understood within psychiatry?

Psychosis defines a mental state characterized by impaired reality testing. Individuals in a psychotic state infer incorrectly about reality and are unable to determine the accuracy of their own thoughts and perceptions. They are unable to change their minds even if presented with contrary evidence (Sadock & Sadock, 2000). Although associations with various biological parameters have been made or inferred (e.g., at the level of neurotransmitters, brain structure, or functioning), *psychosis* is a term used clinically. It denotes the expression of abnormal beliefs (delusions), abnormal sensory experiences (hallucinations) and/or thought disorder. *Delusions* are themselves defined as false, unshakable personal ideas or beliefs about the external reality, unshared within the community to which the individual belongs and firmly held despite no (or even obvious contradictory) evidence. *Hallucinations* are defined as false perceptions in the absence of a real external stimulus that are perceived as having the same quality as real perceptions: they are not subject to conscious manipulation and can occur in any sensory modality. Hallucinations may include simple perceptions (such as light, color, taste, and smell) or more complex experiences such as seeing and interacting with fully formed animals and people, hearing voices and composite tactile sensations. *Thought disorder* is a term encompassing disturbance in the *form* of thought, such as loosened associations between (or frank derailment of) the flow of ideas, neologisms, or illogical constructs. Alterations may also be present in the *rate* of a person's speech, such as showing pressure of speech, speaking incessantly, and/or abnormally quickly for that individual. In addition, individuals in a psychotic state may exhibit bizarre or disorganized behavior, become socially withdrawn or unable to carry out their usual activities of daily living. Overarching these experiences is often *lack of insight*, the most common symptom: from the individual's perspective reality is as they are experiencing it—their beliefs and behaviour are not inappropriate to their circumstance. They may well, therefore, not identify themselves as needing help from mental health professionals and, understandably, be bewildered if not angry when others suggest this may be the case.

The use of the term *psychotic* within psychiatry would normally imply a qualitatively different experience from the norm for an individual within their culture. Occasionally hearing voices is a relatively common experience among the general population (Johns & Van Os, 2001) that may be experienced as personally meaningful (e.g., hearing the voice of a deceased loved one) and within many cultures would be understood as a spiritual experience, to be responded to with respect, if not reverence. Psychiatrists would normally be cautious about using the term psychotic to describe such an experience;

someone who occasionally heard voices would not normally need to see a psychiatrist unless they had difficulties extending beyond that. When we use the term "psychosis" as psychiatrists therefore, we're usually invoking the lexicon of mental illness in our understanding of more extreme experience, which would by majority consensus at least be understood as distinctly beyond "normal." Psychosis is not a diagnosis *per se*, however. The term psychosis is not defined in the *International Classification of Diseases* (*ICD-10*) (World Health Organization, 1992) or in the *DSM-V* (American Psychiatric Association, 2013).

In practice, psychosis is most commonly used within psychiatry as an umbrella term for a group of heterogeneous but conceptually and phenomenologically overlapping mental disorders, including schizophrenia, schizophreniform disorder, delusional disorder, schizoaffective disorder, and affective psychoses (e.g., bipolar disorder). Psychosis here is understood to be the end point of a complex interplay of our genes, environment, and experience, with the relative contribution of those factors unique to the individual. Although each woman's journey into psychosis will be unique, for many women, medication often has significant, if not transformative, life-saving benefit. That is not the case for everyone however, and such benefit is not necessarily without cost, given the experience of sometimes considerable side effects. Of particular concern for many women is firstly the potential for weight gain with many antipsychotic medications and secondly the cessation of menstruation (via reversible elevation of prolactin hormone), which compromises fertility and increases risk of osteoporosis longer-term.

The term psychosis may also be used more loosely to describe significant difficulties with the integration or full awareness of experience that might be described as "dissociation," sometimes seen in women who have diagnoses of borderline personality disorder, many of whom experienced early life trauma. In this context, it's not unusual for women to describe hearing critical voices of others (e.g., telling them to harm themselves). These voices might usefully be thought about as fragments of earlier lived experiences, painfully resonating still in the present. Whether heard literally as those past abusive individuals or otherwise, these experiences are often described by psychiatrists as "pseudo-psychotic" to differentiate them from the psychotic "illnesses" described above (i.e., schizophrenia, bipolar disorder, etc.). Prescribing of antipsychotic medication here is a contentious area, subject to cultural prescribing practice, individual clinician view, and the relationship dynamics that can arise between any individual patient and doctor. In our experience, when the active processes driving psychotic symptoms appear to be primarily psychological, medication is often ineffective, other than possibly providing nonspecific benefit (such as improved sleep or reduction of anxiety levels) and/or on a psychological level as a vehicle for a woman to experience care and concern from her doctor, if the prescription of medication has that symbolic value for her.

Lastly, the term psychosis within psychiatry may also be used to describe symptoms in "organic" states of brain dysfunction, such as the confusion of delirium, the acute intoxication of drug use or its withdrawal, or the impairment of consciousness and its reflective capacity in dementia. Psychotic symptoms within this group usually remit if the underlying organic cause itself can be successfully treated.

CURRENT RESEARCH PERSPECTIVES WITHIN PSYCHIATRY

Do symptom profiles and outcomes differ among men and women with psychosis?

Somewhat surprisingly given the uncertainty regarding etiology, pathogenesis and treatment of psychotic illnesses, differences between the sexes are one of the most consistently reported findings (Kraepelin, 1904; Kretschmer, 1936; Abel, Drake, & Goldstein, 2010). Indeed, differences in age of onset, symptomatology, and course of illness can differentiate women and men suffering from psychosis and may influence the outcome of their treatment (Canuso & Pandina, 2007; Diflorio & Jones, 2010). These distinct characteristics have been accounted for alternatively as the product of a distinct biological milieu, variations in specific neurobiological structures, or social and psychosocial factors; only recently have they been conceptualized as the outcome of the interplay of biological and psychosocial influences (Leung & Chue, 2000; Canuso & Pandina, 2007). Before clarifying clinical features in more detail, it is important to clarify the conceptual and clinical distinctions between bipolar disorder and schizophrenia.

The historical division of psychotic disorder into schizophrenia ("non-affective" i.e., not mood related) and manic-depressive ("affective") illness derives from the extensive clinical work of Emil Kraepelin at the end of the nineteenth century. Kraepelin considered patients to be suffering from dementia praecox (later defined schizophrenia by Eugen Bleuler) and manic-depressive psychosis (bipolar disorder). The former applied when the patient was suffering from a long-term deteriorating condition; the latter when the patient was having distinct episodes of illness alternated with periods of normal functioning. Although modern classification divides these entities assuming they reflect distinct etiologies, different forms of psychosis have been also placed on a continuum of symptom severity and function impairment raging from affective to non-affective disorders, with schizophrenia at the most severe end of the spectrum and bipolar disorder at the least severe (Crow 1986). Recently, both the dichotomous and the continuum views have been challenged by clinical and neurobiological studies, showing both overlaps and distinctions between affective and non-affective psychosis. A plausible model to explain similarities and differences between schizophrenia and bipolar disorder should consider both common and unique risk factors. According to this model, certain susceptibility genes, shared by both disorders, may constitute a risk for psychosis in general, and the specific type of disorder developed may be the consequence of environmental exposure as well as genetic predisposition (Murray et al., 2004). This approach may be useful to explain a consistent difference between women and men that emerges when the epidemiology (incidence and distribution) of these conditions is considered. Women are less likely to receive a diagnosis of non-affective psychosis than men while they have the same likelihood of being diagnosed with an affective psychotic disorder (Canuso & Pandina, 2007; Jogia, Dima, & Frangou, 2012). Nonetheless, in both affective and non-affective psychosis (e.g., schizophrenia and bipolar disorder) women tend to have a later age of onset than men (Bardenstein & McGlashan, 1990; Grant et al., 2005).

The majority of the studies in schizophrenia and schizophrenia-like disorders strongly suggest that women and men can be differentiated on the basis of their symptom profile. Women are more likely to present auditory hallucinations, persecutory delusions, paranoia, and delusions of reference in the context of more marked mood symptoms (e.g., low mood) or pronounced anxiety. Moreover, these symptoms tend to vary more over time due to the menstrual cycle, increasing their intensity in the luteal phase and decreasing when the level of oestrogens are higher (follicular phase)[1] (Leung & Chue, 2000; Canuso & Pandina, 2007). The potential significance of oestrogen is discussed more below. Research in first episode psychosis (which has the advantage of not being confounded by the longer-term impact of biological, psychological or social factors associated with the illness or its treatment) has also started to show a predominance for positive symptoms (e.g., delusions, hallucinations) in women when compared to men, who conversely show more lethargy, apathy, and withdrawal from social activities.

Significantly, these clinical characteristics described above are also thought to be associated with better outcomes in women with schizophrenia and schizophrenia-like disorders, mostly explained as the consequence of better school and work functioning, better social network, and ability to engage with care than men (Canuso & Pandina, 2007; Diflorio & Jones, 2010; Cotton et al., 2013). Again these findings among those with chronic illness are echoed by research in first episode psychosis, where an overall more negative prognosis in men has been found (Canuso & Pandina, 2007; Jogia et al., 2012).

Despite a less consistent body of evidence, women with bipolar disorder also seem to report delusions and hallucinations more often than men (Brunig, Sarkar, Effenberger, Schoofs, & Kruger, 2009; L. V. Kessing, 2008; L. V. Kessing, 2004). Unlike the evidence for schizophrenia and schizophrenia-like disorders however, studies in individuals with bipolar disorder fail to show a clear difference in prognosis between women and men (Diflorio & Jones, 2010).

How might the same illness be expressed differently between genders?

Another not mutually exclusive hypothesis would consider the role that social factors have in modelling the expression of a disease. Notably, when men and women are affected by the same illnesses, its expression, the way they describe it, and the symptoms they report, tend to differ. For example, women are inclined to have more atypical (under-threshold), cyclical psychotic symptoms with a more marked affective component, and this has been linked with less diagnostic concordance for women than men (Leung & Chue, 2000); therefore, the later age of onset of psychosis in women may be the result of difficulties in recognizing and diagnosing the disorder, especially since the present diagnostic criteria are based on studies with an excess of male participants (Leening et al., 2014; Hamilton, Galdas, & Essex, 2015). The differences observed in affective and non-affective psychosis between women and men can be, at least in part, the result of the interplay of distinct hormonal milieus and social and psychosocial characteristics. Indeed, women with psychosis have higher levels of social support and a more close network of relationships than men and this seems to be the result of a more intense pressure to socialize and share emotions (Barajas, Ochoa, Obiols, & Lalucat-Jo, 2015). Furthermore, women are more likely to feel "appreciated or supported" by their friends and family members and feel that they can "open up" to their friends and family members than men. These results may highlight the importance of psychosocial interventions for this population (Salokangas et al., 2013).

Interestingly, the same social factors seem to modulate the differential impact of childhood trauma, one of the most important risk factors for psychosis, in men and women. Generally, subjects with severe psychiatric disorders are more likely to have experienced more frequent and more severe early adversities and psychological difficulties than people without past or current mental conditions (Mauritz et al., 2013). This is particularly true in the case of psychosis. Varese et al. (2012) have shown that case-controlled, cross-sectional as well as prospective studies are consistent in reporting odds ratios between 2.75 and 2.99 of developing psychosis in adulthood in individuals who suffered physical, sexual, emotional abuse and physical or emotional neglect in childhood. Furthermore, early-life adversity is associated with specific clinical characteristics of patients in depression, bipolar disorder, and psychosis in a dose-response fashion (Lang et al. 2004; Heim et al. 2010; Putnam et al. 2010; Larsson et al. 2013; Berg et al. 2014). Although this effect is present in men as well as women, childhood trauma may associate with a different symptom profile depending on gender (Garcia et al., 2016). Greater exposure to childhood adversities is significantly associated with more positive and negative psychotic symptoms as well as an overall poorer functionality, but only in women (Garcia et al., 2016). Similar to what has been shown for the general symptom profiles in men and women with psychosis, the negative impact of childhood trauma in women, but not in men, is magnified when there is an absence of social support (Gayer-Anderson et al., 2015). This is even more important considering that women are more commonly exposed to abuse than men, as has been shown in numerous studies, following the seminal study from Felitti et al. 1998 where, in a representative U.S. sample of 17,337 participants, there was a prevalence of 10.6 percent for emotional abuse (women 13.1 percent and men 7.6 percent), 28.3 percent physical abuse (women 27.0 percent and men 29.9 percent), 20.7 percent sexual abuse (women 24.7 percent and men 16.0 percent), emotional neglect 14.8 percent (women 16.7 percent and men 12.4 percent), and physical neglect 9.9 percent (women 9.2 percent and 10.8 percent).

Are men's and women's brains biologically different in health and illness?

From a biological point of view, women's and men's brains are exposed to a different hormonal environment throughout their lifespan. This has consequences on the structure of the brain, with a well-defined sexual dimorphism of the adult brain and also on the different patterns of alterations associate with psychosis in both sexes. Women are characterized by larger volumes, relative to cerebrum size, particularly in frontal and medial paralimbic cortices (Goldstein et al., 2001). Furthermore, women have higher neuronal density, number of gyri and an overall more complex brain surface than men, especially in the frontal regions (Lüders et al. 2002; Ruigrok et al. 2014). Finally, oestrogens are thought to moderate the effect of the main stress hormones (i.e., glucocorticoids and catecholamine) on neuronal architecture. Indeed they have been shown to modulate the neuronal cycle and to influence the magnitude of cortisol secretion (i.e., higher in the luteal phase) (Bale, 2015).

Differences in brain structure are also present in women and men with psychotic disorders, with these differences present in non-affective psychosis more clearly than in affective psychosis. Despite some inconsistencies, it has been shown that women with schizophrenia have more sparse and less severe structural brain abnormalities than men with the illness (Canuso & Pandina, 2007). Enlarged ventricles, decreased temporal lobe volumes, decreased volume in language associated regions, and more asymmetries in the planum temporalis are more likely to be found in men with non-affective psychosis than women (McDonald et al., 2000; Canuso & Pandina, 2007). The same pattern (more severe brain abnormalities in men than women), even though to a lesser extent, is reported in affective psychosis. Indeed men with the disorder show greater abnormalities in the ventral pre-frontal cortex, amygdala and hippocampal complex (Jogia et al., 2012).

WHAT ROLE MIGHT HORMONES PLAY?

The onset of illness

The difference in age of onset for psychotic illness between the sexes is in line with the widespread, but still poorly elucidated, notion that oestrogens might play a protective role against stress and diseases throughout the lifespan (Gale and Gillespie, 2001; Mozaffarian et al., 2015). Indeed, women are less inclined than men to develop health conditions in which stress and inflammation are aetiologically important or acknowledged risk factors, such as cardiovascular diseases and diabetes (Gale and Gillespie, 2001; Mozaffarian et al., 2015). As environmental stressors are pivotal in the development of a psychiatric disorder, oestrogen may help the individual to adjust and react to the exposure to stressors (e.g., physical and sexual abuse) known to increase the risk of psychosis (Morgan & Fisher, 2007; Duchesne & Pruessner, 2013). This may help clarify why women are characterized by a preponderance of late-onset schizophrenia, typically in the years immediately before or after menopause, when there is a drop in the oestrogen production (Falkenburg & Tracy, 2014). Conversely, in women with schizophrenia, the age at onset is inversely related with the age of menarche, suggesting that longer exposure to oestrogens can defer the onset of psychosis (Cohen, Seeman, Gotowiec, & Kopala, 1999).

The expression of illness

Oestrogens have shown to have a modulatory function on different neurotransmitter systems; particularly, they appear to have anti-dopaminergic effect in the striatum and dopamine is thought to be central in facilitating psychotic experiences (Di Paolo, 1994). This may help explain the variation of symptom intensity often reported in women depending on the phase on the menstrual cycle (see above; Canuso & Pandina, 2007). Unfortunately, whether an anti-dopaminergic effect by oestrogens is present in women with psychosis, and if this interaction plays a role in symptom management, is still unclear (Canuso & Pandina, 2007).

Response to treatment

Undoubtedly, women are more likely to achieve a more rapid treatment response with lower doses of antipsychotics than men (Lindamer, Lohr, Harris, & Jeste, 2004; van der Leeuw et al., 2013). That said, older women show a worse treatment response than both their younger counterparts and older men (Canuso & Pandina, 2007). One explanation here could be that among younger women, the better response to medication is a result of being more likely to take medication as prescribed, but then changes in oestrogen activity as women age leads to declining biological responsiveness to the medication. One might argue by contrast that this is simply a behavioral change on behalf of women, (i.e., being less likely to conform to expectations of medication concordance as they age). Intriguingly, however, and supporting a more biological account here at least, when the efficacy of different second-generation antipsychotics has been tested there is no indication of a gender effect. Indeed risperidone, olanzapine, and quetiapine appear to have the same efficacy in both women and men with psychosis, while clozapine appears to be more slightly effective in men (Canuso & Pandina, 2007). As atypical antipsychotics have a higher affinity for the serotonin 5-HT$_{2A}$ relative to dopamine, it is possible that oestrogens do not add a significant benefit to the overall antipsychotic efficacy as they are mainly active on dopamine (Canuso & Pandina, 2007). Another confounding factor is the influence that antipsychotics have on prolactin. This hormone, influencing the rhythmic production of oestrogens, is important in regulating the menstrual cycle. As antipsychotics increase its concentration, they can determine menstrual cycle irregularities, reducing the protective effect of oestrogens (Canuso & Pandina, 2007).

Increasingly, research has shown the importance of gender in the interplay of biological and psychosocial factors in the expression of disease, influencing age of onset, clinical presentation, course of illness, and response to treatment. Despite the nature of the relationships between these different factors remaining undetermined, holding these different explanatory factors and models in mind during the clinical encounter offers an unparalleled opportunity to better understand women's experiences and provide better support and treatment.

THREE CASE STUDIES

On our National Health Service (NHS) mental health unit in South London, UK, the majority of the women (aged between 18–65 years) have diagnoses of psychotic illness (namely bipolar disorder, schizophrenia, or schizoaffective disorder). Many have a history of early life trauma and have had repeated loss and/or abuse as recurring themes throughout their adult lives. The majority have been compulsorily detained in hospital against their will under the UK's Mental Health Act, with the criteria for admission being suspected or established mental disorder associated with a perceived level of risk to self and/or others that cannot be safely contained or addressed within the community. For admission to be deemed necessary, all community options will have been exhausted. It must be noted, therefore, that these cases provide examples of more severe illness/disturbance, lesser degrees of which would not necessitate hospital admission and would be routinely supported by community interventions and treatment.

For the purposes of confidentiality, the following case studies are amalgams. They are not, therefore, stories of three specific women but rather stories woven from different women's accounts, sufficiently changed in detail throughout to be unidentifiable to any one specific individual.

Case study 1: Helen

Helen is a 62-year-old, retired, white British music teacher who lives alone. Born and brought up in Scotland, her parents, now deceased, were both Polish immigrants. She has a sister who lives some hours away; they occasionally speak on the phone and see each other at Christmas. She has no children and describes herself as a life-long single, bar one unconsummated relationship with a man in her early twenties. She is not known to have experienced any trauma in early life; her development and early years appear to have been unremarkable. She had no significant mental or physical health problems until her mid-forties, when she first came into contact with mental health services. She is a practicing Catholic, regularly attending church but avoiding participating in the church community. In recent years, she appears to have very limited social engagement or interests otherwise.

At the time of her first presentation to services, Helen had approached her primary-care physician concerned that for some time her neighbors were poisoning her water supply; she reported knowing this as her hair felt brittle and her skin unusually dry. She was referred to a community mental health team and after assessment this belief was understood to be delusional; she was diagnosed with a "delusional disorder" on the basis that this belief appeared circumscribed and she denied any other symptoms of psychosis or major affective illness. In discussion with both Helen and, with her permission, her sister via telephone, there appeared to be no clear precipitant to her illness. Whilst Helen rejected professionals' explanation of delusional thinking, she agreed to take an antipsychotic medication on the basis that it might help her chronic insomnia. She repeatedly declined to see a psychologist. By her account, she took the medication consistently for a year and it did help her sleep to some extent. During this time her concerns about her neighbors completely abated. She continued to assert she had no problems with her mental health, however, and said on reflection she thought perhaps there had been a more general problem with the local water supply as she had read something in the newspaper suggesting this may have been the case. Throughout, she managed to continue working as a music teacher and her difficulties were seemingly unknown to colleagues or friends. After a year taking medication, she and her psychiatrist agreed she would stop it on the basis she appeared very well. This had been her first episode of illness and, most importantly, she was very keen to stop medication given the side effects she had experienced that she found difficult to tolerate, in particular weight gain. She recounted feeling "not herself" as she had always prided herself on her slim figure and was disturbed to gradually find most items in her wardrobe no longer fitted. She was subsequently discharged back to primary care. Helen had no contact with mental health services for three years subsequently and was understood to have remained very well and still working without any medication.

Helen was re-referred by primary care when her beliefs about her neighbors returned. This occurred around the time of increasing stress at work. Over the following four years, despite resumption of medication treatment and some (albeit limited) engagement in psychological therapy, these beliefs became more elaborate and she meanwhile became increasingly preoccupied with the belief that female colleagues at work were conspiring against her due, she believed, to jealousy over the fact that a senior male colleague found her attractive. In addition, she described other experiences, such as hearing her neighbors and colleagues talking about her, including across distances of some miles. These experiences were understood to be auditory hallucinations. Her diagnosis was changed to that of schizophrenia. On three occasions, she was compulsorily admitted to mental health units after each time presenting herself to Accident & Emergency departments in a distressed state, requesting assistance for physical health problems due to others poisoning her. She always declined voluntary admission, continuing to assert she had no mental health problems. During these periods in hospital, her beliefs and auditory hallucinations also abated with treatment, however, over time she lost her employment, became reliant on state benefits, and appeared to lose contact with former friends and colleagues.

Over recent years and now in her sixties, Helen's illness has evolved further. Despite taking medication, she is understood to spend most of her daily life preoccupied by a complex delusional system, in which she believes she is the rightful wife of a television celebrity, denied her status due to a conspiracy orchestrated by the imposter in her place. This knowledge came to her as a revelatory moment when watching this celebrity on television. She experienced herself in direct eye contact with him and, through his expression, knew he was secretly signaling their unique connection. Since that time, she has experienced daily, routine communication with him, hearing his voice directly talking to her via the radio and telephone wires in the street; she also frequently interprets overhead airplanes as signaling his love. She writes letters to him in response, care of his agent, and writes regularly to various politicians about her situation, expressing concern for his welfare in convoluted, at times difficult, to follow language (understood as the symptom of "thought disorder"). Most days she goes to cafés local to the television studio, believing he knows she does so to show him her support. She has never approached the celebrity in person and does not appear to know his home address.

Occasionally, Helen becomes troubled (although not obviously distressed) by the resurgence of ideas concerning neighbors poisoning her. She's also at times convinced that people have come into her property at night and moved items around; on occasion, they've replaced things such as her fridge or cooker with similar but not identical versions. She can't say who would do this, or why, but she has been sufficiently concerned about her safety that on occasion she has spent the night in her car. She has continued to have repeated compulsory admissions to mental health units when her delusionally driven behavior has increased to the point she is deemed more vulnerable, such as when local police have come across her sleeping in her car at night or when she has come to the attention of armed police by her attempts to enter secure areas of parliament to petition politicians in person about her situation regarding the celebrity.

When exploring the internal consistency of her belief system, Helen's thought processes seem to become vague and her explanations circular; she is perplexed by any detailed questioning as, for her, the truth of her claims are self-evident. In the context of the reality she experiences, she does not appear to dwell on the apparently surprising state of affairs regarding the television celebrity. Neither does she appear particularly emotional when discussing it, to that extent her beliefs and associated mood could be described as "emotionally incongruent," also a recognized feature of schizophrenia. Most of the time she reports feeling well and reasonably content, alluding confidently to a time in future when she will take her rightful place at the celebrity's side. She manages her day-to-day affairs, is always immaculately dressed, and carries herself with great dignity in her interactions with staff. Historically, she has always politely but firmly resisted attempts to address her "social inclusion" (e.g., to engage her with local day centers, voluntary work, or other social activities) as she has no wish to explore how else she might spend her time. She has rejected all attempts to engage her in any kind of psychological therapy to explore her experiences, their potential meaning for her, and how she manages or might manage them. From both her self-report and professionals' observation, she appears satisfied with the quality of her life.

Regarding ongoing treatment, Helen's psychiatrist has the sense that Helen is humoring her when she agrees to take medication and that she sees health professionals as essentially benign but misguided. Her psychiatrist acknowledges that, from Helen's perspective, all treatment is completely unnecessary as she does not have a mental health problem, and meanwhile Helen's experience in recent years has been that medication does not change what she believes or hears which, for Helen, confirms her experiences are indeed real. She laughs politely when referring to the fact she and health professionals have to "agree to disagree" about the nature of her experiences. She appears happy to see her community mental health nurse and psychiatrist on a regular basis for reviews. It remains unclear to what extent Helen avoids active confrontation with health professionals due to her personality, cultural background (in regard to her gender also), illness (i.e., incongruity between beliefs, mood, action), or out of a pragmatism borne of years of repeated periods of compulsory detention—or possibly a combination of all these factors.

Although medication now doesn't fundamentally change Helen's beliefs or experiences, taking an overview of her functioning it does appear that when taking medication consistently she is less driven to act out on her beliefs, e.g., during periods of taking medication she doesn't try and get into parliament and she doesn't appear concerned by other paranoid beliefs such as being poisoned. That said, given the ongoing intensity of her delusional experiences even whilst on medication, her psychiatrist remains concerned that there is only a small margin of benefit in taking medication, given the risk of side effects in terms of her physical health. Helen's sister has meanwhile contacted services to express her anger and disbelief that Helen is "allowed" to continue living independently, given the number of times she has had urgent phone calls from services, in particular the police, concerned about Helen's vulnerability (e.g., as a woman sleeping in her car when she's been more paranoid about her neighbors). She says she "always worries something terrible will happen" and has threatened to take legal action against the mental health team. Helen herself is very clear she loves her home of many years, has no wish to move, and appears horrified by the idea of sheltered accommodation with staff support. For now, mental health services are hoping that Helen will continue to voluntarily accept medication in the community, and in doing so will maintain a fragile stability whereby she can maintain her independence in her own home for as long as she wishes to do so.

Case 2: Alice

Alice is a 26-year-old white English woman with a history of growing up in a large, wealthy but emotionally austere family environment. After travelling and volunteering in Africa for a year following school, she returned to the UK and completed a degree in Global Health. Over the course of her undergraduate studies, she suffered two significant periods of depression during which she was treated within primary care with a combination of antidepressants and psychotherapy. These episodes were understood respectively to have been precipitated by an abusive relationship and the death by suicide of her older brother, who had a significant substance misuse problem.

Alice first came into contact with secondary mental health care during her first year in postgraduate studies in International Development. Against a background of gradually worsening sleep for some weeks, over a period of days her behavior had become uncharacteristically disturbed: she was highly argumentative with her flatmates, sent sexually explicit emails to her supervisor, and posted an online profile in which she claimed she was CEO of a charity she'd set up to found an orphanage in Africa. Things came to a head one night when she brought home three men she didn't know but had met on the street. One of these men made an unwanted sexual advance toward one of her flatmates; during the ensuing row, Alice picked up a kitchen knife and threatened to cut her own throat. Another flatmate disarmed her, an ambulance was called, and she was taken to the Accident & Emergency department of her local hospital, accompanied by her friends who told staff how concerned they were about the recent changes in her behavior. From there, she was assessed by mental health professionals and compulsorily detained to a mental health unit.

Alice's admission to hospital was initially very difficult. She was in ongoing conflict with staff over her detention and the need to take any medication, only taking a small amount of the medication prescribed and strongly asserting it was unnecessary as she was not mentally unwell. She repeatedly insisted she be allowed to leave immediately as she was needed on important international humanitarian business, claiming she'd been emailed by several world leaders urgently requesting her help. She was increasingly sexually disinhibited with some staff and verbally abusive to others. On the third day of her admission, staff insisted on removing her mobile phone after another patient alerted them that she had taken photographs of staff and patients and posted them online; at this point she attempted to assault staff, furious that her phone had been taken from her. Both the nursing and medical team attempted to verbally de-escalate the situation, but dialogue proved impossible as she was intensely distressed, screaming staff were "pedophiles," and spitting at and attempting to hit them. As she was still refusing oral medication, the staff team decided it was necessary to physically restrain her to administer sedative medication by intramuscular injection. A group of seven nurses and healthcare assistants (male and female) took her in arm-holds to the de-escalation room on the ward, where she continued to refuse oral medication. Staff held her against resistance in the standard restraint position on the mattress in the room and a female nurse gave her a dose of short-acting sedative medication by injection. She became calmer over the following thirty minutes and then slept for a couple of hours. Later that day she very reluctantly agreed to start regular oral medication (an antipsychotic/anti-manic oral medication agent combined with a benzodiazepine). This medication was increased over the following days. Gradually, her sleep improved, levels of arousal lessened as did her disinhibition. Over the following two weeks, she became less acutely confrontational and demanding with staff, no longer insisting she was the CEO of a charity, although she remained labile in mood, appearing elated, singing and dancing on the ward at times, tearful at others.

Over the following three weeks, Alice started to go off the ward for periods, with staff at first, then unaccompanied, as her mood and sleep continued to stabilize. With support of friends, her family, and hospital staff she began to repair relationships and took down posts and photographs she had made online whilst unwell. In discussion with her psychiatrist, she rejected the diagnosis of a manic episode of bipolar affective disorder. Whilst she recognized things had felt "a bit out of control" before admission, she insisted her detention wasn't justified and in particular staff had "overreacted" when they restrained her and gave her an injection against her will. She described feeling very distressed by this event, in particular the presence of male staff physically restraining her, referring to memories of a past traumatic event that she did not wish to detail. She made a formal complaint to the hospital about this. She declined to discuss her behavior or presentation when she was more unwell in any detail, stating she just wanted to focus on "looking to the future" and getting out of hospital; it wasn't clear to what extent she might not be able to recall everything that had happened, was choosing not to, or simply didn't want to discuss it with the psychiatrist in question.

Alice described feeling "much less stressed" as the admission progressed, but remained ambivalent about the role of hospital treatment in her improvement. She continued to take medication only reluctantly, not least due to experiencing significant side effects, including some weight gain and muscular tiredness. In addition, her menstruation stopped and she was found to have a high prolactin hormone level (due to the medication). She felt very disturbed by the cessation of her menstrual periods and cited it as evidence of how unnatural taking medication was. She was also concerned that it might prevent her getting pregnant, something she said was "on her list" alongside finding a partner in the next few years. Her medication was switched to an alternative in view of this, and her prolactin level began to fall. She saw the ward psychologist on three occasions, which she did say was helpful, and also engaged with the ward occupational therapist, who supported her in liaising with her college regarding her return to her studies.

Six weeks later, at the point of discharge to initially intensive community support, Alice appeared fully well. Her relationship with her psychiatrist, whilst superficially friendly, remained strained, however: Alice spoke freely about past depression, but was uncomfortable with what she called being "labelled with bipolar," and having read up online, preferred to simply refer to having had a "period of elevated mood," which she attributed to the strain of her studies and tensions with her flatmates. She remained adamant early in the admission she should not have been restrained to be given medication against her will, which she maintained was an abusive act that resonated with past personal trauma. She also felt the psychiatrist's strong advice to continue medication to avoid risking relapse did not accommodate her preference to be medication-free and rely only on natural remedies, which she planned to do. She was keen to return to her course full-time immediately and distance herself from mental health services, rejecting the psychiatrist's advice she return to her studies more slowly whilst continuing follow-up with her community mental health team. She did, however, agree to re-engage with the psychotherapist she saw and trusted previously in the community and to see her primary care doctor for follow-up, including for a repeat blood test of her prolactin levels. To date, a year later she has had no further contact with mental health services as far as the team is aware.

Case 3: Janet

Janet is a 45-year-old, morbidly obese black British woman of mixed Jamaican and British heritage. She lives alone. She has a disabled mother, four sisters, and a brother all living in neighboring areas but she sees them infrequently, bar one sister who visits intermittently when Janet is in hospital. Janet is not known to have ever had a relationship and has no children. Although Janet worked for some years as an administrator after leaving school, since her mid-twenties she has not worked and has had repeated admissions to hospital with a diagnosis of initially bipolar disorder, then schizophrenia, and more recently, schizoaffective disorder.

In the past, Janet had admissions to a mental health unit every couple of years or so, each time for a couple of months; over the last two years she has had four admissions to hospital, each time her discharge back home has broken down rapidly despite increasing levels of community support. The role of medication here is not entirely clear; she has not missed her depot medication outside of hospital, but each time has stopped her oral tablet mood stabilizer, she has become unwell again. Each admission has been precipitated by a member of the public seeing Janet disturbed in a public place, and subsequently calling emergency services. On the most recent occasion, less than a week after discharge (at which point she appeared well and confident about plans to go home) she was found sitting in her nightdress at a bus stop at 2 a.m.

When in hospital, Janet's admissions have been characterized by an initial period of florid, seemingly profoundly psychotic disturbance with a marked affective (mood) component. When most disturbed, her thoughts appear very disorganized, she is highly abusive (in particularly racially abusive to African staff) and she speaks in fragmented terms about spirits and demons, referring to spirits interfering with her in some way, including coming through doors to visit her, although the nature of this experience has been difficult to clarify given her disorganized dialogue and interaction. Her behavior at these times is chaotic; she will urinate and defecate on her bedroom floor, walk naked in the ward corridor, and walk into ward therapeutic groups gesticulating angrily and haranguing staff for their incompetence with a tirade of expletives. These periods of profound disturbance last for a few weeks, gradually her presentation and behavior stabilizes, but she will spend many weeks still irritable, intermittently racist, and generally insistent staff attend to her needs immediately. These themes remain, although with much less intensity, as she makes further progress and starts to spend periods of time off the ward by herself each day. Her engagement with others remains limited throughout her time in hospital, she spends long periods in the lounge watching TV but doesn't socialize or engage in small talk with patients or staff. She rarely attends therapeutic groups but does goes to the consultant psychiatrist and OT's weekly group; however, in the group she appears to struggle to engage in dialogue, usually asserting her presence through odd behavior such as loudly praying with her eyes tightly shut, or if silent and seemingly not feeling attended to, she will leave.

There is particular running tension between Janet and nursing staff over her self-care. She will insist, for example, that staff obtain large incontinence pads for her, otherwise, she will publicly urinate on the floor. She views it as staff responsibly then to clean up after her, including removing soiled pads from her bedroom cupboard where she chooses to dispose of them (rather than in the bathroom facility). Given an overview of her health, medical and nursing staff view her as capable of using the bathroom and buying her own sanitary wear if she wishes.

The demands of Janet's care, practically and also emotionally withstanding her abuse, has caused considerable strain amongst the nursing team and they have repeatedly discussed this in the staff reflective practice group (supervised by an external psychotherapist facilitator). Janet has also, on more than one occasion, been the subject of a dedicated case discussion group with the ward psychologist, where staff have discussed the challenges in her care and how they might respond to them in ways that would feel more helpful. During these discussions, staff have noted Janet's need for care feels as if it were at the most basic mothering level, as if she were an infant.

Although Janet has refused to see the ward psychologist herself, she has seen a trainee psychologist on one occasion for the purposes of an audit of trauma in relation to BMI (body mass index). During that research interview, she disclosed a past history of childhood sexual abuse that she declined subsequently to discuss further.

Janet has always appeared keen on her weekly face-to-face review with her (female) consultant psychiatrist even when at her most disturbed. At those times, she will speak angrily and shout in jumbled terms that are difficult to follow but weave around themes of her being abused by staff and Africans in particular. She will often also refer to her family and the pressures her mother puts her under, although it's thought her mother is not actively involved in her life at all (and hasn't been for years). It has never proved possible to really think with her about pressure she might currently feel now including within her relationships with staff and her psychiatrist. Given the apparent level of hostility toward her psychiatrist at these times, it can feel surprisingly difficult to end the interview, and Janet will appear reluctant to leave the room with the psychiatrist eventually standing, holding the door open, and encouraging her to leave. As two-way dialogue becomes more possible, when challenged about her behavior, however gently, Janet will immediately become highly defensive and maintain the problem is simply that others are incompetent, uncaring, and abusive; she remains adamant she is only a victim of others' aggression and lack of care. Trying to suggest to her that, whilst it's recognized that this may have been her experience in the past, might it be something that could be thought more about in the here-and-now?—has not yet proved fruitful. When the past or her relationships are mentioned, she habitually changes the topic and talks pressingly of other matters. Janet will also often refer to herself as "schizophrenic" or "bipolar," but it's not proved possible to think with her what she means by those terms herself, beyond what seems to be her implied assertion that these labels in themselves are explanatory and indicate others should be caring for her. On occasion, the psychiatrist has observed the surprising rapidity of her readmissions, and tried to think with her about why they have occurred. Janet has insisted others, such as her support workers, have not visited when they should have done but has quickly changed the subject. The psychiatrist has also attempted to speculate with her that it might be difficult to be on her own in the flat, after the noise and company of the ward, and has wondered with her whether she might feel lonely back at home and perhaps bored with little to do. Janet has always firmly insisted she is fully occupied in her time attending to the practicalities of life and meanwhile has no need for friends, saying she is someone who is happy with her own company and "doesn't need other people." Touching on these matters is always fleeting, as Janet will quickly divert onto other topics. These discussions tend to leave her psychiatrist feeling somewhat controlled and defeated by these interactions, which always remain on territory Janet appears comfortable on, namely the failings of others and sorting practical matters such as rent. Janet has again recently been discharged, much to her apparent and seemingly somewhat triumphant satisfaction, but with her psychiatrist remaining concerned history will again repeat itself and she will continue to be admitted under similar circumstances, which, to date, the team has yet to find what feels like a helpful therapeutic response to, i.e., one that might support change. Ultimately, this apparent failure might reflect a disconnect between the ambitions and priorities of the health team and Janet herself.

The case studies in overview

For a treating psychiatrist, Helen and Alice represent women with psychotic illnesses that can, to some degree at least, be circumscribed and understood within an illness paradigm. The route to illness has been seemingly more complicated in the case of Alice, where her difficulties appear to have been shaped to some degree in part, if not actually precipitated by, difficult life experiences that will resonate for many women along gender lines. Their response to treatment is also markedly different—Alice comes into hospital very unwell, but this episode of her life appears to be just that—an episode—and one from which potentially she may recover completely, never to return a similar state of mind again; although given the severity of her difficulties on this occasion one might speculate some degree of significant mental health difficulties may reemerge for her again in life—most likely at times of interpersonal stress, social difficulty, or physical health challenge. Helen is however, from the outside at least, less fortunate. Her illness is now no longer significantly changed by medication, perhaps in part speaking to the declining response to treatment associated with aging for women, speculatively due to oestrogen changes mentioned earlier in this chapter. One might argue that a negative view of her quality of life now in relation to illness at best over-simplifies and at worst is patronizing, unjustifiably appropriating an individual woman's experience—as gendered constructions of normality have historically done.

The case of Janet is clinically far more complex and illustrates the impossibility sometimes of knowing to what degree someone is unwell in the sense of having an illness (which of course also speaks to the complexity of what we mean by "illness," and who decides that), or to what degree their disturbance can be explained as a manifestation of their personality in the context of ongoing emotional difficulties or turmoil, perhaps too great to be consciously experienced directly and thereby expressed and on some level discharged through behavior in interaction with others. The most that health professionals and the hospital institutions themselves in these situations can do sometimes is to metaphorically (and literally at times) hold a woman to keep her safe and contain that disturbance and distress until some aspects of their experience can be talked and thought about, sufficient for seemingly sometimes disconnected aspects of their psyche to "re-group" to allow them to reemerge into the reality of outside the world, at which point in the community they will accept whatever treatment or support they feel ready or inclined to do. The relative importance of different treatment modalities such as medication or specific psychological therapy available on the ward may not always be clear for some women who present with diagnostic challenges such as Janet, and often one has a sense that allowing time is the most important aspect of healing, allowing a woman to "get herself together." In turn, the greatest challenge at times, especially when a woman's admission can feel highly emotionally charged, is to avoid actual harm to a woman through our interventions, whether that be related to specific treatments, potentially unhelpful responses of staff, or the broader experience for a woman of being institutionalized, with all the loss of control that can involve, resonating as it may with past trauma.

WOMEN'S EXPERIENCES OF THE WARD

Whilst the ward has a psychologist and a variety of therapeutic groups (including music and art therapy), most of the women on our ward with diagnoses of psychotic illness would normally be under compulsion to take antipsychotic medication as a key component of their treatment, and as the case of Alice illustrates, this is often the most contentious aspect of an admission. The majority of women are understood to have some degree of a positive response to medication during their stay in hospital, which usually lasts between one to three months, and most leave feeling and appearing much better than on admission. This said, it is not uncommon for women to leave hospital remaining uncomfortable about the use of an illness framework to understand their difficulties and ambivalent about their treatment, often maintaining that whilst things may have been difficult before admission in some way, their detention was unnecessary. It is often implied, if not explicit, they will stop medication once home and no longer compelled to take it. Notwithstanding this unresolved tension, by discharge women often report aspects of hospital care—whether that is general support from the nurses, the occupational therapist, psychologist, or hospital social work team—as helpful, and something they are thankful for. By the time of discharge, their perspective can often feel like that of Helen's, (i.e., that staff are essentially benign but misguided). For some women, their relationship with our unit is an ongoing and complex one over time, with periods of managing independently in the community interspersed with repeated compulsory admissions usually after they have stopped their medication and the cycle of illness has returned.

As the case of Janet illustrates, when women are well and no longer need to be in hospital, it can at that point sometimes feel very difficult to reflect on what has happened and try to learn from it to prevent its repetition. This may be due to "lack of insight" as a feature of their psychosis, i.e., they are not necessarily able to recall, process, and reflect on the reality of everything that transpired when they were at their most unwell or disturbed; they may never recognize they have a mental health problem or accept medication is necessary as a result. But it may also feel more complex, as if in trying to talk about past events one is dragging them back to a traumatic period that, understandably, they wish to seal over and move on from. It can feel helpful sometimes to view long-term serious mental illness, and all the profound loss of health, opportunity, and independence this can bring for a woman, as being akin to a bereavement, that often occurs against a background of other multiples losses, and involves a woman navigating what is commonly (although not unanimously) framed in terms of the stages of grief; i.e., denial, anger, bargaining, depression, and acceptance (Kübler-Ross, 1969), which are often nonlinear and cyclical, and with acceptance (or "insight") a stage that may never be reached.

For the purposes of this chapter, the cases above illustrate the complexity of experience, treatment, and sometimes very difficult balancing of therapeutic good against harm in our setting, where our knowledge and understanding within psychiatry is stretched to its limits on occasion, and pragmatism and hoped-for therapeutic wisdom rather than science can determine decisions. It is not always like that, however. There are many women who, however complex their backgrounds, have more straightforward recoveries and no need for ongoing contact with mental health services when they leave. They may experience one episode of psychotic illness, perhaps in the context of overwhelming emotional stress, and completely recover, never to return. Ultimately, every woman's experience is unique.

STAFF EXPERIENCE OF OUR UNIT

Our ward has been for women patients only for over ten years now, with both male and female staff working on the unit. This switch from being a mixed ward followed a national directive for more gender-sensitive inpatient care. Advertising a consultant psychiatrist post to women-only applications itself caused some controversy at the time. Dissenting voices subsided however, once it was pointed out the potentially problematic nature of men running the ward given that the patients were all women, many with histories of abuse, and in the context of hospital, physically detained on the unit against their will. The fact this needed to be pointed out was in itself interesting.

Over the years, we have found that it is harder to recruit staff to units for women such as ours. Male patients are, anecdotally, more linear in their trajectories of opposition, rising anger, its release, and subsequent relational repair. Although male patients have usually greater physical heft to inflict more significant physical injury to staff, and anecdotally as a group are more prone to explosive violent outbursts, overall nurses often report working in a female environment as more difficult as it tends to be more emotionally draining. It seems as if women who have suffered severe traumas, including the trauma of admission to hospital and having to take medication perhaps against their will, express their hurt, anger, and opposition in more sustained, frequent (albeit possibly "lower grade") acts of verbal and physical aggression, as well as expressing resistance in more passive-aggressive ways that can feel more difficult to openly address and think about. Our ward psychologist who works across the male and female wards, which mirror each other in both layout and function, says the two wards are so different in feel "she can't begin to describe it." In our experience, working only with women has its own challenges—in particular holding in mind the welfare of children under their care and, sometimes, the potentially conflicting interests of a woman as a mother and those of her children. But it can be deeply rewarding and inspiring, as well as full of humor at times. Although gender-based generalizations (about anything) often break down at the level of the individual, the difference in experience for both staff and patients on male and female wards is an area rich for more research and reflection.

IN SUMMARY

From our combined academic and clinical perspectives, our view of psychiatry's role in helping with women with psychosis is to scientifically and clinically continue to try and embrace and understand the complexity. We need to continue to seek to identify predisposing, precipitating, and perpetuating factors for psychosis, be they biological, psychological, or social, and to understand how they relate to each other both at the level of gender for women as a group, and personally for women as individuals with their own unique life stories. We need to continue to name what's helpful to name in terms of manifestations of distress and/or illness, so that we can best communicate shared understandings to effect healing and recovery through the most appropriate means. And we need to continue to develop how we provide gender-based services to best meet the needs of women, in particular in relation to inpatient care, given the challenges that can occur in that context both for patients and staff.

REFERENCES

Abel, K. M., Drake, R., & Goldstein, J. (2010). Sex differences in schizophrenia. *The International Journal of Social Psychiatry*, *22*(5), 417–28. http://doi.org/10.3109/09540261.2010.515205.

American Psychiatric Association. (2013). *DSM-V. American Journal of Psychiatry*. http://doi.org/10.1176/appi.books.9780890425596.744053.

Bale, T. L. (2015). Epigenetic and transgenerational reprogramming of brain development. *Nature Reviews Neuroscience*, *16*(6), 332–44. http://doi.org/10.1038/nrn3818.

Barajas, A., Ochoa, S., Obiols, J. E., & Lalucat-Jo, L. (2015). Gender differences in individuals at high-risk of psychosis: A comprehensive literature review. *Scientific World Journal*, *2015*. http://doi.org/10.1155/2015/430735.

Bardenstein, K. K., & McGlashan, T. H. (1990). Gender differences in affective, schizoaffective, and schizophrenic disorders. A review. *Schizophrenia Research*. http://doi.org/10.1016/0920-9964(90)90034-5.

Berg, a. O., Aas, M., Larsson, S., Nerhus, M., Hauff, E., Andreassen, O. a., & Melle, I. (2014). Childhood trauma mediates the association between ethnic minority status and more severe hallucinations in psychotic disorder. *Psychological Medicine*, *33291714*(1), 1–10. http://doi.org/10.1017/S0033291714001135.

Bräunig, P., Sarkar, R., Effenberger, S., Schoofs, N., & Krüger, S. (2009). Gender differences in psychotic bipolar mania. *Gender Medicine*, *6*(2), 356–61. http://doi.org/10.1016/j.genm.2009.07.004

Canuso, C., & Pandina, G. (2007). Gender and schizophrenia. *Psychopharmacology Bulletin*, *40*, 178–90.

Cohen, R. Z., Seeman, M. V., Gotowiec, A., & Kopala, L. (1999). Earlier puberty as a predictor of later onset of schizophrenia in women. *American Journal of Psychiatry*, *156*(7), 1059–64.

Cotton, S. M., Lambert, M., Berk, M., Schimmelmann, B. G., Butselaar, F. J., McGorry, P. D., & Conus, P. (2013). Gender differences in first episode psychotic mania. *BMC Psychiatry*, *13*, 82. http://doi.org/10.1186/1471-244x-13-82.

Di Paolo, T. (1994). Modulation of brain dopamine transmission by sex steroids. *Reviews in the Neurosciences*, *5*(1), 27–42.

Diflorio, A., & Jones, I. (2010). Is sex important? Gender differences in bipolar disorder. *International Review of Psychiatry (Abingdon, England)*, *22*(5), 437–52. http://doi.org/10.3109/09540261.2010.514601

Duchesne, A., & Pruessner, J. C. (2013). Association between subjective and cortisol stress response depends on the menstrual cycle phase. *Psychoneuroendocrinology*, *38*(12), 3155–59. http://doi.org/10.1016/j.psyneuen.2013.08.009.

Falkenburg, J., & Tracy, D. K. (2014). Sex and schizophrenia: A review of gender differences. *Psychosis: Psychological, Social and Integrative Approaches*, *6*(1), 61–69. http://doi.org/10.1080/17522439.2012.733405.

Felitti, V. J., Anda, R. F., Nordenberg, D., Williamson, D. F., Spitz, A. M., Edwards, V., Marks, J. S. (1998). Relationship of childhood abuse and household dysfunction to many of the leading causes of death in adults: The adverse childhood experiences (ACE) study. *American Journal of Preventive Medicine*, *14*(4), 245–58. http://doi.org/10.1016/S0749-3797(98)00017-8.

Gale, E. a M., & Gillespie, K. M. (2001). Diabetes and gender. *Diabetologia*, *44*(1), 3–15. http://doi.org/10.1007/s001250051573.

Garcia, M., Montalvo, I., Creus, M., Cabezas, Á., Solé, M., Algora, M. J., Labad, J. (2016). Sex differences in the effect of childhood trauma on the clinical expression of early psychosis. *Comprehensive Psychiatry*, *68*, 86–96. http://doi.org/10.1016/j.comppsych.2016.04.004.

Gayer-Anderson, C., Fisher, H. L., Fearon, P., Hutchinson, G., Morgan, K., Dazzan, P., Morgan, C. (2015). Gender differences in the association between childhood physical and sexual abuse, social support and psychosis. *Social Psychiatry and Psychiatric Epidemiology*, *50*(10), 1489–1500. http://doi.org/10.1007/s00127-015-1058-6.

Goldstein, J. M., Seidman, L. J., Horton, N. J., Makris, N., Kennedy, D. N., Caviness, V. S., Tsuang, M. T. (2001). Normal sexual dimorphism of the adult human brain assessed by in vivo magnetic resonance imaging. *Cerebral Cortex*, *11*(6), 490–97. http://doi.org/10.1093/cercor/11.6.490.

Grant, B. F., Stinson, F. S., Hasin, D. S., Dawson, D. A., Chou, S. P., Ruan, W. J., & Huang, B. (2005). Prevalence, Correlates, and Comorbidity of Bipolar I disorder and Axis I and II disorders: Results from the national epidemiologic survey on alcohol and related conditions. *The Journal of Clinical Psychiatry*, \n\t66\n\t(\n\t10\n\t), \n\t1205\n\t-\n\t1215\n\t.

Hamilton, I., Galdas, P., & Essex, H. (2015). Cannabis psychosis, gender matters. *Advances in Dual Diagnosis*, *8*(3), 153–62. http://doi.org/10.1108/ADD-12-2014-0039.

Heim, C., Shugart, M., Craighead, W. E., & Nemeroff, C. B. (2010). Neurobiological and psychiatric consequences of child abuse and neglect. *Developmental Psychobiology*, *52*(7), 671–90. http://doi.org/10.1002/dev.20494.

Jogia, J., Dima, D., & Frangou, S. (2012). Sex differences in bipolar disorder: A review of neuroimaging findings and new evidence. *Bipolar Disorders*, *14*(4), 461–71. http://doi.org/10.1111/j.1399-5618.2012.01014.x.

Johns, L. C., & van Os, J. (2001). The continuity of psychotic experiences in the general population. *Clinical Psychology Review*. http://doi.org/10.1016/S0272-7358(01)00103-9.

Kessing, L. V. (2004). Gender differences in the phenomenology of bipolar disorder. *Bipolar Disorders*, *6*(5), 421–25. http://doi.org/10.1111/j.1399-5618.2004.00135.x.

Kessing, L. V. (2008). The prevalence of mixed episodes during the course of illness in bipolar disorder. *Acta Psychiatrica Scandinavica*, *117*(3), 216–24. http://doi.org/10.1111/j.1600-0447.2007.01131.x.

Kraepelin, E. (1904). Psychiatrie: ein lehrbuch für studirende und aerzte. In *Psychiatrie: ein Lehrbuch für Studirende und Aerzte* (pp. 815–41).

Kretschmer, E. (1936). *Physique and Character, 2nd Ed.* New York: Harcourt, Brace, & Company.

Kübler-Ross, E. (1969). *On death and dying*. New York: Scribner.

Lang, A. J., Stein, M. B., Kennedy, C. M., & Foy, D. W. (2004). Adult psychopathology and intimate partner violence among survivors of childhood maltreatment. *Journal of Interpersonal Violence*, *19*(10), 1102–18. http://doi.org/10.1177/0886260504269090.

Larsson, S., Aas, M., Klungsøyr, O., Agartz, I., Mork, E., Steen, N. E., Lorentzen, S. (2013). Patterns of childhood adverse events are associated with clinical characteristics of bipolar disorder. *BMC Psychiatry*, *13*, 97. http://doi.org/10.1186/1471-244X-13-97.

Leening, M. J. G., Ferket, B. S., Steyerberg, E. W., Kavousi, M., Deckers, J. W., Nieboer, D., … Roos-Hesselink, J. W. (2014). Sex differences in lifetime risk and first manifestation of cardiovascular disease: prospective population based cohort study. *Bmj*, *349*(nov17 9), g5992–g5992. http://doi.org/10.1136/bmj.g5992.

Leung, A., & Chue, P. (2000). Sex differences in schizophrenia, a review of the literature. *Acta Psychiatrica Scandinavica. Supplementum*, *401*, 3–38. http://doi.org/10.1111/j.0065-1591.2000.0ap25.x.

Lindamer, L. A., Lohr, J. B., Harris, M. J., & Jeste, D. V. (2004). Gender, estrogen, and schizophrenia. *Focus*, *2*(1), 138–45. http://doi.org/10.1176/foc.2.1.138.

Lüders, E., Steinmetz, H., & Jäncke, L. (2002). Brain size and grey matter volume in the healthy human brain. *NeuroReport*, *13*(17), 2371–74. http://doi.org/10.1097/01.wnr.0000049603.85580.da.

McDonald, B., Highley, J. R., Walker, M. A., Herron, B. M., Cooper, S. J., Esiri, M. M., & Crow, T. J. (2000). Anomalous asymmetry of fusiform and parahippocampal gyrus gray matter in schizophrenia: A postmortem study. *American Journal of Psychiatry*, *157*(1), 40–47. http://doi.org/10.1176/appi.ajp.157.1.40.

Morgan, C., & Fisher, H. (2007). Environment and schizophrenia: Environmental factors in schizophrenia: Childhood trauma—A critical review. *Schizophrenia Bulletin*, *33*(1), 3–10. http://doi.org/10.1093/schbul/sbl053.

Mozaffarian, D., Benjamin, E. J., Go, a. S., Arnett, D. K., Blaha, M. J., Cushman, M., Turner, M. B. (2015). *Heart Disease and Stroke Statistics—2015 Update: A Report From the American Heart Association*. *Circulation* (Vol. 131). http://doi.org/10.1161/CIR.0000000000000152

Ruigrok, A. N. V, Salimi-khorshidi, G., & Lai, M. (2014). A meta-analysis of sex differences in human brain structure. *Neuroscience and Biobehavioral Reviews*. http://doi.org/10.1016/j.neubiorev.2013.12.004.

Sadock, J., & Sadock, V. A. (2000). Kaplan & Sadock's Comprehensive Textbook of Psychiatry. *Psychiatry Interpersonal and Biological Processes*, *II*, 4884. http://doi.org/10.4067/S0717-92272002000300011.

Salokangas, R. K. R., Nieman, D. H., Heinimaa, M., Svirskis, T., Luutonen, S., From, T., Ruhrmann, S. (2013). Psychosocial outcome in patients at clinical high risk of psychosis: A prospective follow-up. *Social Psychiatry and Psychiatric Epidemiology*. http://doi.org/10.1007/s00127-012-0545-2.

van der Leeuw, C., Habets, P., Gronenschild, E., Domen, P., Michielse, S., van Kroonenburgh, M., Marcelis, M. (2013). Testing the estrogen hypothesis of schizophrenia: Associations between cumulative estrogen exposure and cerebral structural measures. *Schizophrenia Research*, *150*(1), 114–20. http://doi.org/10.1016/j.schres.2013.07.033.

Varese, F., Smeets, F., Drukker, M., Lieverse, R., Lataster, T., Viechtbauer, W., Bentall, R. P. (2012). Childhood adversities increase the risk of psychosis: A meta-analysis of patient-control, prospective-and cross-sectional cohort studies. *Schizophrenia Bulletin*, *38*(4), 661–71. http://doi.org/10.1093/schbul/sbs050.

World Health Organization. (1992). The ICD-10 Classification of Mental and Behavioural Disorders. *International Classification*, *10*, 1–267.

NOTE

1. The menstrual cycle can be divided in two successive phases on the basis of an alternatively higher concentration of estrogen (follicular phase) and progesterone (luteal phase).

Chapter Nine

Schizophrenia in Women as Compared to Men

Theories to Help Explain the Difference

Mary V. Seeman

Although more contested than any other diagnostic category in psychiatry, no exploration of women and psychosis would be complete without a discussion of schizophrenia, the many factors that are thought to contribute to its symptoms, the many reported gender differences, and the main treatment implications that arise from these differences. This chapter is based on papers selected from biopsychosocial databases for the years 1990–2016. The following search terms were used in interaction with "schizophrenia": brain, childbirth, course, gender, genes, hormones, immunity, menopause, menstruation, onset, outcome, parenting, postpartum, pregnancy, prodrome, symptoms, treatment. Not all relevant papers could be cited, so a selection was made on the basis of currency, readability, comprehensiveness, and uniqueness. The main findings were that, although both women and men suffer from symptoms that fit the current diagnostic classification of schizophrenia, there are important gender differences in the timing of onset, course of illness, nature of symptoms, and response to treatment. The exact reasons for these differences are not known but there are many theories, many of which are addressed in the course of the chapter.

EPIDEMIOLOGY

The diagnosis of schizophrenia is applied more frequently to men than to women, the ratio being approximately 1.4/1 (Bao & Swaab, 2010). The peak age of onset of frank psychotic symptoms (hallucinations and delusions) is 20–24 years in men and three to five years later in women (Aleman, Kahn, & Selten, 2003; Castle Sham, & Murray, 1998; Eranti et al., 2013). Until the fourth decade of life, men receive a schizophrenia diagnosis more often than women (Bao & Swaab, 2010). Subsequently, the reported incidence in women begins to rise in direct association, it is thought, with a decline in circulating levels of gonadal hormones (Häfner, 2003; Halbreich & Kahn, 2003). Late-onset schizophrenia (i.e., after age 40) is up to ten times more common in women than in men (Howard et al., 1993; Meesters et al., 2012).

When compared to men diagnosed with schizophrenia, women are more likely to be employed (Marwaha & Johnson, 2004). Thus, as a group, they enjoy a relatively higher standard of living. They are less likely to end their lives by suicide, although suicide in the context of schizophrenia is a danger for both sexes (Seeman, 2009a). Women are more likely than men to marry and have children (Seeman, 2010), which means more affective ties but added responsibilities. Women are less likely than men to be charged with crimes or to spend time in prison (Carlström & Långström, 2009), thus defying the public's automatic association of mental illness with dangerousness. Women are less likely than their male counterparts to ever be homeless, abuse alcohol or drugs, or refuse recommended treatment (Remington & Seeman, 2015), making them more likely to respond positively to mental health interventions. Women's later onset of symptoms is considered critical to women's generally more favorable course of illness because it gives women time to complete their education, form intimate friendships, and be employed outside the home (Leung & Chue, 2000).

CLINICAL FEATURES

There is evidence that women who develop schizophrenia symptoms not only have a later onset of illness than men but that they also have fewer and less severe premorbid psychological problems (whether motor, cognitive, social, affective, or academic) (Allen et al., 2013). During the prodromal period, men and women, to an equal extent, exhibit school problems, appear preoccupied with one or more "overvalued" ideas (most frequently philosophical, supernatural or moral) and report feelings of unreality and of "something being wrong" (Möller & Husby, 2000). Withdrawal from friends and family during the prodrome is less marked in young women than in young men (Möller & Husby, 2000). An acute onset of psychotic symptoms, which is independently associated with a better prognosis, is more common in women, whereas a more gradual onset is more common in men (Moriarty et al., 2001).

Because initial psychotic symptoms are often acute and short-lived in women, they may delay seeking treatment (Cohen, Gotowiec, & Seeman, 2000). Another explanation for the delay is that women's relatively larger and more supportive social networks (Seeman, 1982) may be able, for a time, to contain the distress. It is also possible that the behavioral manifestations of schizophrenia in young women are less disturbing to family and society than those of more violence-prone men (Seeman, 1982) so that family members do not rush to bring them to treatment.

With respect to the clinical features once illness starts, women show more positive symptoms (i.e., hallucinations and delusions) (Matud, 2004; Rector & Seeman, 1992); women present with fewer negative symptoms (e.g., apathy and social withdrawal) (Maric et al., 2003), less severe cognitive symptoms (Krysta et al., 2013), but more prominent affective features (Willhite et al., 2008). Women are usually described as experiencing a less chronic course of illness (Moriarty et al., 2001). The gender differences in negative and cognitive symptoms are believed to result from males' comparatively greater exposure to fetal stress, obstetrical trauma, brain trauma during childhood and exposure to toxic substances during adolescence (Remington & Seeman, 2015). The gender difference in emotional expressiveness seen in schizophrenia has also been noted in the general population (Chaplin, 2015). Women with this diagnosis tend not only to show more affect than male peers; they also experience a more acute onset of illness and a more intermittent course of illness (Röttig et al., 2004). Perhaps as a result, women are more often than men diagnosed with schizoaffective disorder (Röttig et al., 2004).

In women, the relative lack of negative symptoms (considered a hallmark of schizophrenia, since positive and cognitive symptoms are present in essentially all forms of psychosis) and the presence of affective symptoms (a hallmark of mood disorder) present a diagnostic challenge, sometimes resulting in a delay in antipsychotic treatment (Cascio et al., 2012). This is a potential disadvantage for women because many believe that early intervention leads to better long-term outcomes (Harvey, Lepage, & Malla, 2007; McGorry et al., 2009). The connection between an early start to treatment (both pharmacological and psychological) and improved outcome remains controversial (Harrigan, McGorry, et al., 2003) because early treatment, while attenuating symptoms, exposes individuals to a stigmatized diagnostic label. Moreover, the original rationale for early treatment—the belief that psychosis is toxic to the brain—has never been proven. Evidence for and against early treatment is bedevilled by terms whose meaning is imprecise, such as "early," "intervention," and "outcome" (Davidson and McGlashan, 1997). A recent prospective study suggests that diverse, multidisciplinary community-based psychosocial interventions improve one-year outcomes in early psychosis (Na et al., 2016). Another recent study found that a combination of engagement in a specialized program and adherence to medication improves positive and negative symptoms and results in a superior functional outcome at twelve, twenty-four, and thirty-six months (Golay et al., 2016). Attribution of success to the treatment is premature, however, because treatment adherence is rarely monitored in studies of the effects of early intervention.

GENDER DIFFERENCES IN RISK FACTORS FOR SCHIZOPHRENIA

Individual psychosocial and biological risk factors have been identified for schizophrenia but, in life, risks work in concert with one another and the boundary between biological, psychological and social is illusory. For both women and men, a history of schizophrenia in the family heightens the risk for a personal diagnosis of a similar condition (Esterberg et al., 2010). Advanced paternal age is another potential risk factor that affects both sexes equally, age potentially causing DNA mutations in the father's sperm that contribute to risk (McGrath et al., 2014; Rosenfield et al., 2010). Being born in winter or spring has been associated with subsequent schizophrenia, less often in women than in men (Martínez-Ortega et al., 2011). It is not clear why there should be a sex difference except that male fetuses are more vulnerable than female fetuses to adversity in whatever form, excess viral exposure during winter and early spring being an example of adversity (Fineberg et al., 2016; Wells, 2000). The relative invulnerability of female fetuses is an early female advantage but, since frail male fetuses succumb early, males who manage to survive may, on average, be biologically hardier that females (Sandman, Glynn, & Davis, 2013).

Trauma in childhood, both psychological and physical, is associated with high activity levels and with risk-taking, both qualities linked to masculinity. In fact, boys are twice as likely as girls to suffer brain injury (Orlovska et al., 2014), which may increase schizophrenia risk, especially for those with a family history of psychosis (AbdelMalik et al., 2003). Additional risk factors for both genders in childhood are sexual and emotional trauma, as well as severe neglect and psychosocial adversity (Arsenault et al., 2011; Morgan & Fisher, 2007; Read et al., 2005; Varese et al., 2012). Preliminary evidence suggests that the risk of psychosis following childhood sexual abuse is higher in women than in men (Bebbington et al., 2011; Conus et al., 2010; Cutajar et al., 2010; Fisher et al., 2009), a connection that may be modifiable by the degree of available social support (Gayer-Anderson et al., 2015).

Substance abuse is another known risk factor for schizophrenia that is less prevalent in females than in males (Zilberman et al., 2003). The risk-taking trait, closely associated as previously stated with masculinity, leads to more and earlier experimentation with substances (Zilberman et al., 2003). The relative risk is complicated, however, by the fact that women's substance-related problems are "telescoped," meaning that women, though they drink alcohol or use drugs less often than men, suffer the health sequelae sooner (Hernandez-Avila, Rounsaville, & Kranzler, 2004). Cannabis is the substance that has been receiving the most attention recently as a potential trigger to schizophrenia. A recent study measuring brain glucose metabolism using positron emission tomography in cannabis abusers has suggested that women are more sensitive than men to the adverse effects of cannabis on the brain (Wiers et al., 2016).

An excess of premorbid risk factors may be the explanation for the earlier onset of schizophrenia in men relative to women, with the consequence that education may be truncated in men with schizophrenia (Seeman, 1982). In general, men with early schizophrenia also face a greater likelihood of family upheaval and experience less emotional closeness to family members than women do, which subsequently leads to difficulty in establishing intimate relationships (Seeman, 1982). Perhaps for such reasons, men with this diagnosis are less likely than women to marry. In women with schizophrenia, a later onset of symptoms, uninterrupted schooling and a pre-illness work history assist in finding employment after diagnosis. Such factors help to raise self-esteem as well as the standard of living; they also lower the likelihood of criminal activity (Marhawa & Johnson, 2004). Finding employment in Western countries is less difficult for women diagnosed with schizophrenia than for men not only because of women's later age of illness onset but also because there are more entry-level jobs for women than there are for men (Marhawa & Johnson, 2004).

Expectations may also differ depending on culture. Families may expect less of their daughters than of their sons with regard to academic, financial, athletic, and social success (Barcellos et al., 2014; Varner & Mandara, 2013). The extra parental pressure exerted on sons may contribute to the stress that brings forward the onset age of psychosis in men and ultimately leads to a better prognosis for women (Remington & Seeman, 2015). There are, of course, other culturally-determined pressures on women, for instance, the pressure to please, to be thin, to nurture, to provide child care, to be fertile. Gender-specific pressures can be important in preventing or delaying recovery. Gender-specific pressures can also lead to gender-specific delusions in schizophrenia, such as the denial of pregnancy (Nau et al., 2011) or delusional pregnancy (Seeman, 2014).

HORMONAL EXPLANATORY MECHANISMS

Many mechanisms have been advanced to account for the various male/ female differences in schizophrenia (Seeman, 2009b), among which are hormonal mechanisms (Allen, Purves-Tyson, & Weickert, 2015; Gleich, Deijen, & Drent, 2014; Hara et al., 2015). Estradiol in particular is known to be involved in the growth of neurons, in the formation of synapses between nerve cells, in the branching out of dendrites, and in nerve cell myelination, all of which contribute to brain plasticity, the resilience factor that helps to fight off injury and dysfunction. Estrogens also interact with brain neurotransmitters (Barth, Villringer, & Sacher, 2015). Both estrogen and progesterone receptors are expressed throughout brain regions (especially the amygdala and the hippocampus) that control affect and cognition, two brain processes that are severely affected by schizophrenia (Barth, Villringer, & Sacher, 2015). These receptors allow local hormones to effect change in cells that are responsible for the release of a variety of neurotransmitters. Female hormones, for this reason, have been called neuroprotective (Seeman & Lang, 1990). One particularly important mechanism of protection against psychotic symptoms is through the impact of estrogen on dopamine neurotransmission (its synthesis, release, turnover, and degradation), since dopamine is thought to play an important role in the molecular biology of schizophrenia (Di Paolo, 1994). Another vital function of estrogens is to protect against stress (Albert, Pruessner, & Newhouse, 2015), which is assumed to play a major role in triggering schizophrenic symptoms. Yet another very significant function may be an epigenetic one—controlling which schizophrenia-related genes are expressed and which are silenced (McCarthy et al., 2009).

Because a woman's lifespan is characterized by major hormonal transition periods marked by rising estrogen levels during puberty, high estrogen levels during pregnancy, and rapid falls postpartum, as well as by declining levels during the menopausal transition and low levels after menopause, symptoms of schizophrenia in women vary accordingly, partly explaining their intermittent pattern throughout reproductive life and their gradual worsening during the transition to menopause (Seeman, 2012a; Seeman, 2012b). This understanding has led to an important treatment advance: the adjunctive use of estrogen or selective estrogen receptor modulators to the medication regimen of patients with schizophrenia (Kulkarni, Hayes, & Gavrilidis, 2012; Kulkarni et al., 2008) for the amelioration of both psychotic and cognitive symptoms (Herringa et al., 2015; Weickert, Allen, & Weickert, 2016).

Although hormones remain critical in explaining gender differences in schizophrenia, immune factors are receiving increasing attention (Khandaker et al., 2015) because many aspects of immunity markedly differ in men and women, women usually showing a more pronounced immune response than men (Pennell, Galligan, & Fish, 2012). Whole genome searches have revealed many DNA sites that are seen more often in those with this diagnosis than in the general population, but one of the strongest schizophrenia associations is with the area on chromosome 6 that houses genes responsible for immunity (Schizophrenia Working Group, 2014). Very recent interest has centered on a gene that makes proteins that help antibodies fight off bacteria and other foreign substances. That same gene is thought to be also responsible for triggering the start of nerve cell pruning that takes place in the brain during adolescence (Sekar et al., 2016). It has been hypothesized that a particular form of this gene goes into overdrive in individuals with schizophrenia (Sekar et al., 2016), over-trimming neurons and, in this way, giving birth to clinical symptoms. Interestingly, the timing and rate of synaptic pruning during adolescence have been known to differ between the sexes. This difference has been attributed to hormones (De Bellis et al., 2001), but may, in fact, be attributable to factors related to immunology.

GENDER DIFFERENCES IN BRAIN PATHOLOGY

Over the years, many sex differences have been found in the brains of individuals with schizophrenia (Goldstein et al., 2007; Gur et al., 2004; Womer et al., 2016) but it is far from clear how these differences translate into the increased prevalence of schizophrenia in males or the later onset age in women or the sex-specific nature of symptoms in schizophrenia. Male/female structural differences in the brain become apparent in adolescence, the very time of synaptic pruning and of first appearance of classical schizophrenia symptoms (Giedd et al., 2012; Lenroot & Giedd, 2010). Controlling for body size, the male brain is about 10 percent larger in volume than the female brain (Giedd et al., 2012; Lenroot & Giedd, 2010), and males reach peak volumes chronologically later than females (Giedd et al., 2012; Lenroot & Giedd, 2010). Because of the gender difference in the rate of growth of many brain regions, the results of measurements of size differences depend on the age at which they are measured, which accounts for the variability of results. Concordance is greatest for the following gender size: a larger caudate and hippocampus in females; a larger amygdala in males. Size may (or may not) dictate function.

GENDER DIFFERENCES IN PREVENTION AND TREATMENT

Prevention and treatment of schizophrenia can be considered on a population or community (macro) level, or a family and individual (micro) level. Prevention on a macro level would include abolition of poverty, an end to discrimination against minorities, the elimination of mental illness stigma, the reduction of societal violence, the availability of universal parental education and prenatal support, and routine child and adolescent mental health screening (Schwartz & Meyer, 2010). Such measures might reduce the incidence of mental illnesses such as schizophrenia in both sexes, although poverty, violence, and stigma may affect women and men differently. Stigma is a powerful example. Violence is seen in both men and women with schizophrenia (Rice et al., 2015) but men are stigmatized as being more dangerous. Women with schizophrenia, on the other hand, are stigmatized as unfit parents (Dolman, Jones, & Howard, 2013; Krumm et al., 2014). In former years, they were often sterilized (Gamble, 1948). Nowadays, women with schizophrenia too often lose custody of their children (Seeman, 2012c). The police and criminal justice systems are overly harsh with the men (Teplin, 1990) while health and residential systems neglect the safety of women with schizophrenia and their children (Copperman & Knowles, 2006; Kidd et al., 2013; Waddell et al., 2006).

Micro prevention includes parenting support programs for mothers with schizophrenia (Bhatia et al., 2004). These are social and educational services that provide support and respite when needed, and that teach parenting skills to help children of mentally ill parents flourish (Gladstone et al., 2014; Krumm, Becker, & Wiegand-Grefe, 2013; Seeman, 2012c). Family interventions assist in instances of domestic abuse in families (Jonas et al., 2014). Individual level interventions that especially benefit women include addressing sexual abuse, domestic abuse, contraception, menstrual cycles, pregnancy, labor and delivery, breast-feeding, and menopause (Seeman, 2012 a & b; Seeman, 2013; Seeman & Gupta, 2013; Seeman & Ross, 2011). Specially tailored interventions may be necessary for lesbian and transgender women who suffer from schizophrenia (Seeman, 2015). Newly immigrant women who develop schizophrenia require services geared to their special needs such as interpreter services and liaison services with appropriate ethnic and religious communities (Yakushko et al., 2008); elderly women require special attention to drug doses geared to their age and health status (Chernomas et al., 2000). Although these are necessary services for male immigrants and elderly men as well, specific attention must be paid to gender differences (e.g., interpreter services for immigrant mothers with mental illness and drug dose differences related to age and gender). The pharmacokinetics and pharmacodynamics of antipsychotic drug treatment differ in men and women because of differences in body size, lipid composition, liver enzyme activity, and smoking habits, among other metabolic and behavioral contrasts. This means that, on average, women require lower doses of these drugs than men do (Seeman, 1989; Smith, 2010; Usall et al., 2007). The choice of specific drugs and doses needs to be modulated according to both sex and age (Franconi et al., 2007), and attention paid to adverse effects that affect one sex preferentially. Examples include sexual difficulties, hormonal problems, sedation that interferes with childcare responsibilities, osteoporosis, and risk of breast and prostate cancer (Haack et al., 2009; Seeman, 2009b). Women are said to experience adverse effects to a greater degree than men, including a higher prevalence of weight gain, type 2 diabetes, osteoporosis, and specific cardiovascular complications (e.g. *torsades de pointes*), in addition to complications of pregnancy (Seeman, 2009c). Drug treatment may be required during pregnancy and breastfeeding. As a consequence, the medical prescription of drugs that are relatively safe for the fetus and neonate is an issue of particular concern to women (Gentile, 2004).

Women diagnosed with schizophrenia are reported to respond more readily and more fully to medical treatment than their male counterparts and to require comparatively lower doses of antipsychotic medication to achieve symptom control (Smith, 2010; Usall et al., 2007). Women also respond better on average than men to psychological treatments (Brabban, Tai, & Turkington, 2009). Women's superior response to medical intervention may be explained by a faithful adherence to medical regimens and therapy protocols (Miller, 2015), and to superior social supports, the existence of close others who endorse, encourage, and enforce care interventions. In contrast to men with schizophrenia and due perhaps to a relatively intact premorbid state and a relatively late onset of illness, women with a schizophrenia diagnosis often maintain supportive social networks throughout the course of illness, which helps buffer the burden of schizophrenia.

CONCLUSION

Schizophrenia, although a contested diagnosis, is generally considered to be one of the most serious mental illnesses, with an exceptionally adverse impact on quality of life (Awad & Voruganti, 2016). It affects the patient, the patient's family and the community in which the patient lives. Schizophrenia is not an equal opportunity illness; it affects some persons much more severely than others. On average, women are less severely affected than men, but this generalization comes with many caveats. The diagnosis is often made late in women, robbing them of the advantage of an early start to effective treatment (Häfner et al., 2013). Women with schizophrenia are often the victims of abuse (Jonas et al., 2014). Although they require lower doses of antipsychotics than men in order to manage their symptoms, they are often treated with textbook doses (as determined by clinical trials conducted with men) and thus experience unnecessary side effects (Seeman, 2009c). Clinical services often overlook women's specific needs (Seeman & Gupta, 2013) and treat women as they do men. Gender differences in schizophrenia are important because they can guide clinicians toward gender-specific treatments that promise greater safety and greater effectiveness for both genders. An important lesson of gender differences is the realization that psychosis manifests itself differently in different persons and that its treatment needs to be individually-oriented and individually-tailored for maximal benefit.

REFERENCES

AbdelMalik, P., Husted, J., Chow, E. W., & Bassett, A. S. (2003). Childhood head injury and expression of schizophrenia in multiply affected families. *Archives of General Psychiatry* 60, 231–36.

Alameda, L., Golay, P., Baumann, P. S., Ferrari, C., Do, K. Q., & Conus, P. (2016). Age at the time of exposure to trauma modulates the psychopathological profile in patients with early psychosis. *Journal of Clinical Psychiatry* 77, e612–18.

Albert, K., Pruessner, J., & Newhouse, P. (2015). Estradiol levels modulate brain activity and negative responses to psychosocial stress across the menstrual cycle. *Psychoneuroendocrinology*, 59, 14–24.

Aleman, A., Kahn, R. S., & Selten, J.-P. (2003). Sex differences in the risk of schizophrenia: evidence from meta-analysis. *Archives of General Psychiatry*, 60, 565–71.

Allen, D.N., Strauss, G. P., Barchard, K. A., Vertinski, M., Carpenter, W. T., & Buchanan, R. W. (2013). Changes in academic and social premorbid adjustment across sex and developmental period in individuals with schizophrenia. *Schizophrenia Research* 146, 132–37.

Allen, K. M., Purves-Tyson, T. D., & Weickert, C. S. (2015). Reproductive hormones and schizophrenia. *Schizophrenia Research* 168, 601–02.

Arseneault, L., Cannon, M., Fisher, H. L., Polanczyk, G., Mott, T. E., & Caspi, A. (2011). Childhood trauma and children's emerging psychotic symptoms: a genetically sensitive longitudinal cohort study. *American Journal of Psychiatry* 168, 65–72.

Awad A. G. & Voruganti L. N. P. (eds.) (2016). *Beyond assessment of quality of life in schizophrenia*. Springer International Publishing, Switzerland.

Bao, A. M., & Swaab, D. F. (2010). Sex differences in the brain, behavior, and neuropsychiatric disorders. *Neuroscientist* 16, 550–65.

Barcellos, S. H., Carvalho, L. S., & Lleras-Muney, A. (2014). Child gender and parental investments in India: Are boys and girls treated differently? *American Economic Journal: Applied Economics* 6, 157–89.

Barth, C., Villringer, A., Sacher, J. (2015). Sex hormones affect neurotransmitters and shape the adult female brain during hormonal transition periods. *Frontiers in Neuroscience* doi: 10.3389/fnins.2015.00037.

Bebbington, P., Jonas, S., Kuipers, E., King, M., Cooper, C., Brugha, T., Meltzer, H., McManus, S., & Jenkins, R. (2011). Childhood sexual abuse and psychosis: data from a cross-sectional national psychiatric survey in England. *British Journal of Psychiatry* 199, 29–37.

Bhatia, T., Franzos, M. A., Wood, J. A., Nimgaonkar, V. L., & Deshpande, S.N. (2004). Gender and procreation among patients with schizophrenia. *Schizophrenia Research* 68, 387–94.

Brabban, A., Tai, S., & Turkington, D. (2009). Predictors of outcome in brief cognitive behavior therapy for schizophrenia. *Schizophrenia Bulletin* 35, 859–64.

Carlström, S. F., Långström, P. L. (2009). Risk factors for violent crime in schizophrenia: a national cohort study of 13,806 patients. *Journal of Clinical Psychiatry* 2009 70, 362–69.

Cascio, M. T., Cella, M., Preti, A., Meneghelli, A., & Cocchi, A. (2012). Gender and duration of untreated psychosis: a systematic review and meta-analysis. *Early Intervention in Psychiatry* 6, 115–27.

Castle, D., Sham, P., & Murray, R. (1998). Differences in distribution of ages of onset in males and females with schizophrenia. *Schizophrenia Research* 33, 179–83.

Chaplin, T. M. (2015). Gender and emotion expression: A developmental contextual perspective. *Emotion Review* 7, 14–21.

Chernomas, W. M., Clarke, D. E. & Chisholm, F. A. (2000). Perspectives of women living with schizophrenia. *Psychiatric Services* 51, 1517–21.

Cohen, R. Z., Gotowiec, A., & Seeman, M. V. (2000). Duration of pretreatment phases in schizophrenia: women and men. *Canadian Journal of Psychiatry* 45, 544–47.

Conus, P., Cotton, S., Schimmelmann, B. G., McGorry, P. D., & Lambert, M. (2010). Pretreatment and outcome correlates of sexual and physical trauma in an epidemiological cohort of first-episode psychosis patients. *Schizophrenia Bulletin* 36, 1105–14.

Copperman, J., & Knowles, K. (2006). Developing women only and gender sensitive practices in inpatient wards—current issues and challenges. *Journal of Adult Protection* 8, 15–30.

Cutajar, M. C., Mullen, P. E., Ogloff, J. R. P., Thomas, S., Wells, D. L., & Spataro, J. (2010). Schizophrenia and other psychotic disorders in a cohort of sexually abused children. *Archives of General Psychiatry* 67, 1114–19.

Davidson, L. & McGlashan, T.H. (1997). The varied outcomes of schizophrenia. *Canadian Journal of Psychiatry* 42, 34–43.

De Bellis, M. D., Keshavan, M. S., Beers, S. R., Hall, J., Frustaci, K., Masalehdan, A., Noll, J., & Boring, A. M. (2001). Sex differences in brain maturation during childhood and adolescence. *Cerebral Cortex* 11, 552–57.

Di Paolo, T. (1994). Modulation of brain dopamine transmission by sex steroids. *Review of Neuroscience* 5, 27–41.

Dolman, C., Jones, I., & Howard, L. M. (2013) Pre-conception to parenting: A systematic review and meta-synthesis of the qualitative literature on motherhood for women with severe mental illness. *Archives of Womens Mental Health*, 16, 173–96.

Eranti, S. V., MacCabe, J. H., Bundy, H. & Murray, R. M. (2013). Gender difference in age at onset of schizophrenia: a meta-analysis. *Psychological Medicine* 43, 155–67.

Esterberg, M. L., Trotman, H. D., Holtzman, C., Compton, M. T., & Walker, E. F. (2010). The impact of a family history of psychosis on age-at-onset and positive and negative symptoms of schizophrenia: a meta-analysis. *Schizophrenia Research,* 120, 121–30.

Fineberg, A. M., Ellman, L. M., Schaefer, C. A., Maxwell, S. D., Shen, L., Chaudhury, N. H., Cook, A. L., Bresnahan, M. A., Susser, E. S., & Brown A. S. (2016). Fetal exposure to maternal stress and risk for schizophrenia spectrum disorders among offspring: Differential influences of fetal sex. *Psychiatry Research* 236, 91–97.

Fisher, H. L., Morgan, C., Dazzan, P., Craig, T. K., Morgan, K., Hutchinson, G., Jones, P. B., Doody, G. A., Pariante, C., McGuffin, P., Murray, R. M., Leff, J., & Fearon, P. (2009). Gender differences in the association between childhood abuse and psychosis. *British Journal of Psychiatry* 194, 319–25.

Franconi, F., Brunelleschi, S., Steardo, L., & Cuomo, V. (2007). Gender differences in drug responses. *Pharmacological Research* 55, 81–95.

Gamble, C. J. (1948). The sterilization of psychotic patients under state laws. *American Journal of Psychiatry* 105:60–62.

Gayer-Anderson, C., Fisher, H. L., Fearon, P. Hutchinson, G., Morgan, K., Dazzan, P., Boydell, J., Doody, GA., Jones, P. B., Murray, R. M., Craig, T. K., & Morgan, C. (2015). Gender differences in the association between childhood physical and sexual abuse, social support and psychosis. *Social Psychiatry and Psychiatric Epidemiology* 50, 1489–500.

Gentile, S. (2004). Clinical utilization of atypical antipsychotics in pregnancy and lactation. *Annals of Pharmacotherapy*, 38, 1265–271.

Giedd, J. N., Raznahan, A., Mills, K. L. & Lenroot, R. K. (2012). Review: magnetic resonance imaging of male/female differences in human adolescent brain anatomy. *Biology of Sex Differences* 3, 19. 9 pages.

Gladstone, B. M., Boydell, K. M., Seeman, M. V., & McKeever, P. (2014). Analysis of a support group for children of parents with mental illnesses: Managing stressful situations. *Qualitative Health Research* 24, 1171–82.

Gleich, T., Deijen, J. B., & Drent, M. L. (2014). The involvement of the hypothalamic-pituitary- gonadal, hypothalamic-pituitary-adrenal and somatotrophic axes in the development and treatment of schizophrenia. SDI Paper Template Version 1.6 Date 11.10.2012.

Golay, P., Alameda, L., Baumann, P., Elowe, J., Progin, P., Polari, A., & Conus, P. (2016). Duration of untreated psychosis: Impact of the definition of treatment onset on its predictive value over three years of treatment. *Journal of Psychiatric Research* 77, 15–21.

Goldstein, J. M., Seidman, L. J., Makris, N., Ahern, T., O'Brien, L. M., Caviness Jr., V. S., Kennedy, D. N., Faraone, S. V., & Tsuang, M. T. (2007). Hypothalamic abnormalities in schizophrenia: sex effects and genetic vulnerability. *Biological Psychiatry*, 61, 935–45.

Gur, R. E., Kohler, C., Turetsky, B. I., Siegel, S. J., Kanes, S. J., Bilker, W. B., Brennan, A. R., & Gur, R. C. (2004). A sexually dimorphic ratio of orbitofrontal to amygdala volume is altered in schizophrenia. *Biological Psychiatry* 55, 512–17.

Haack, S., Seeringer, A., Thurmann, P.A., Becker, T., & Kirchheiner, J. (2009). Sex-specific differences in side effects of psychotropic drugs: genes or gender? *Pharmacogenomics* 10, 1511–15.

Häfner, H. (2003). Gender differences in schizophrenia. *Psychoneuroendocrinology* 28(Suppl 2), 17–54.

Häfner, H., Maurer K., & W. an der Heiden W. (2013). ABC Schizophrenia study: an overview of results since 1996. *Social Psychiatry and Psychiatric Epidemiology* 48, 1021–31.

Halbreich, U., & Kahn, L.S. (2003). Hormonal aspects of schizophrenias: An overview. *Psychoneuroendocrinology* 28 (Suppl. 2), 1–16.

Hara, Y., Waters, E. M., McEwen, B. S., & Morrison, J. H. (2015). Estrogen effects on cognitive and synaptic health over the lifecourse. *Physiological Reviews* 95, 785–807.

Harrigan, S. M., McGorry, P. D., & Krstev, H. (2003) Does treatment delay in first-episode psychosis really matter? *Psychological Medicine* 33 97–110.

Harvey, P., Lepage, M., & Malla, A. (2007). Benefits of enriched intervention compared with standard care for patients with recent-onset psychosis: a metaanalytic approach. *Canadian Journal of Psychiatry* 52, 464–72.

Hernandez-Avila, C. A., Rounsaville, B. J., & Kranzler, H. R. (2004). Opioid-, cannabis-and alcohol-dependent women show more rapid progression to substance abuse treatment. *Drug and Alcohol Dependence* 74, 265–72.

Herringa, S. M., Bergemann, M. J. H., Goverde, A. J., & Sommer, I. E. (2015). Sex hormones and oxytocin augmentation strategies in schizophrenia: A quantitative review. *Schizophrenia Research* 168, 603–13.

Howard, R., Castle, D., Wessley, S., & Murray, R. (1993). Differences in late- and early-onset schizophrenia. *American Journal of Psychiatry* 150, 846–47.

Jonas, S., Khalifeh, H., Bebbington, P.E., McManus, S., Brugha, T., Meltzer H., & Howard L. M. (2014). Gender differences in intimate partner violence and psychiatric disorders in England: Results from the 2007 adult psychiatric morbidity survey. *Epidemiology and Psychiatric Sciences* 23, 189–99.

Khandaker, G. M., Cousins, L., Deakin, J., Lennox, B. R., Yolken, R., & Jones, P. B. (2015). Inflammation and immunity in schizophrenia: Implications for pathophysiology and treatment. *Lancet Psychiatry* 2, 258–70.

Kidd, S. A., Virdee, G., Krupa, T., Burnham, D., Hemingway, D., Margolin, I., Patterson, M., & Zabkiewicz, D. The role of gender in housing for individuals with severe mental illness: A qualitative study of the Canadian service context. *British Medical Journal Open* 2013; 3(6), e002914.

Kirov, G., Jones, P. B., Harvey, I., Lewis, S. W., Toone, B. K., Rifkin, L., Sham, P., & Murray, R.M. (1996). Do obstetric complications cause the earlier age at onset in male than female schizophrenics? *Schizophrenia Research*, 20, 117–24.

Krumm, S., Becker, T., & Wiegand-Grefe, S. (2013). Mental health services for parents affected by mental illness. *Current Opinion in Psychiatry*, 26, 362-368.

Krumm, S., Checchia, C., Badura-Lotter, G., Kilian, R., & Becker, T. (2014). The attitudes of mental health professionals towards patients' desire for children. *BMC Medical Ethics*, 15, 18.

Krysta, K., Murawiec, S., Klasik, A., Wiglusz, M. S., & Krupka-Matuszczyk, I. (2013). Sex-specific differences in cognitive functioning among schizophrenic patients. *Psychiatria Danubina*, 25(Suppl 2), 244–46.

Kulkarni, J., de Castella, A., Fitzgerald, P.B., Gurvich, C.T, Bailey, M., Bartholomeusz, C., & Burger, H. (2008). Estrogen in severe mental illness: A potential new treatment approach. *Archives of General Psychiatry*, 65, 955–60.

Kulkarni, J., Hayes, E., & Gavrilidis, E. (2012). Hormones and schizophrenia. *Current Opinion in Psychiatry*, 25, 89–95.

Lenroot, R. K., & Giedd, J. N. (2010). Sex differences in the adolescent brain. *Brain and Cognition*, 72, 46–55.

Leung. A., & Chue, P. (2000). Sex differences in schizophrenia, a review of the literature. *Acta Psychiatrica Scandinavica*, 101, 3–8.

Marwaha, S., & Johnson, S. (2004). Schizophrenia and employment—a review. *Social Psychiatry and Psychiatric Epidemiology*, 39, 337–49.

Maric, N., Krabbenden, L., Vollebergh, W., de Graaf, R., & van Os, J. (2003). Sex differences in symptoms of psychosis in a non-selected, general population sample. *Schizophrenia Research*, 63, 89–95.

Martínez-Ortega, J. M., Carretero, M. D., Gutiérrez-Rojas, L., Díaz-Atienza, F., Jurado, D., & Gurpegui, M. (2011). Winter birth excess in schizophrenia and in non-schizophrenic psychosis: Sex and birth-cohort differences. *Progress in Neuro-Psychopharmacology & Biological Psychiatry*, 35, 1780–84.

Matud, M. P. (2004). Gender differences in stress and coping styles. *Personality and Individual Differences*, 37, 1401–15.

McCarthy, M., Auger, A. P., Bale, T. L., de Vries, G. J., Dunn, G. A., Forger, N. G., Murray, E. K., Nugent, B. M., Schwarz, J. M., & Wilson, M. E. (2009). The epigenetics of sex differences in the brain. *Journal of Neuroscience* 29, 12815–23.

McGorry P. D., Nelson B., Amminger G. P., Bechdolf A., Francey S. M., Berger G., Riecher-Rössler A., Klosterkötter J., Ruhrmann S., & Schultze-Lutter F. (2009). Intervention in individuals at ultra high risk for psychosis: a review and future directions. *Journal of Clinical Psychiatry 70*, 1206–12.

McGrath, J. J., Petersen, L., Agerbo, E., Mors, O., Mortensen, P. B., & Pedersen, C. B. (2014). A comprehensive assessment of parental age and psychiatric disorders. Journal of the *American Medical Association Psychiatry* 71, 301–09.

Meesters, P. D., de Haan, L., Comijs, H. C., Stek, M. L., Smeets-Janssen, M. M. J., Weeda, M. R., Eikelenboom, P., Smit, J. H., & Beekman, A. T. (2012). Schizophrenia spectrum disorders in later life: Prevalence and distribution of age at onset and sex in a Dutch catchment area. *American Journal of Geriatric Psychiatry* 20, 18–28.

Miller, J. B., Pierce Stiver I. (1997). *The Healing Connection: How Women Form Relationships in Therapy and in Life*. Boston: Beacon Press.

Möller P., & Husby R. (2000). The initial prodrome in schizophrenia: Searching for naturalistic core dimensions of experience and behavior. *Schizophrenia Bulletin* 26, 217–32.

Morgan, C., & Fisher, H. (2007). Environment and schizophrenia: Environmental factors in schizophrenia: Childhood trauma—a critical review. *Schizophrenia Bulletin* 33, 3–10.

Moriarty, P. J., Lieber, D., Bennett, A., White, L., Parrella, M., Harvey, P. D., & Davis, K. L. (2001). Gender differences in poor outcome patients with lifelong schizophrenia. *Schizophrenia Bulletin* 27, 103–13.

Na, E. J., Kang, N. I., Kim, M. Y., Cui, Y., Choi, H. E., Jung, A. J., & Chung, Y. C. (2016). Effects of community mental health service in subjects with early psychosis: One-year prospective follow up. *Community Mental Health Journal* 52, 724–70.

Orlovska, S., Pedersen, M. S., Benros, M. E., Mortensen, P. B., Agerbo, E., & Nordentoft, M. (2014). Head injury as risk factor for psychiatric disorders: A nationwide register-based follow-up study of 113,906 persons with head injury. *American Journal of Psychiatry* 171, 463–69.

Pennell, L. M., Galligan, C. L., & Fish, E. N. (2012). Sex affects immunity. Journal of *Autoimmunity* 38, 282–91.

Read, J., van Os, J., Morrison, A., & Ross, C. A. (2005). Childhood trauma, psychosis and schizophrenia: a literature review with theoretical and clinical implications. *Acta Psychiatrica Scandinavica* 112, 330–50.

Rector, N. A., & Seeman, M. V. (1992). Auditory hallucinations in women and men. *Schizophrenia Research* 7, 233–36.

Reininghaus, U., Gayer-Anderson, C,. Valmaggia, L., Kempton, M. J., Calem, M., Onyejiaka, A., Hubbard, K., Dazzan, P., Beards, S., Fisher, H. L., Mills, J. G., McGuire, P., Craig, T.

K., Garety, P., van Os, J., Murray, R. M., Wykes, T., Myin-Germeys, I., & Morgan, C. (2016) Psychological processes underlying the association between childhood trauma and psychosis in daily life: An experience sampling study. *Psychological Medicine 46*, 2799–813.

Remington, G., & Seeman, M.V. (2015). Schizophrenia and the influence of male gender. *Clinical Pharmacology & Therapeutics 98*, 578–81.

Rice, T., Hoffman, L., & Sher, L. (2015). Portrayal of violent male psychiatric patients by entertainment media and the stigma of psychiatric illness. *Australian and New Zealand Journal of Psychiatry 49*, 849.

Rosenfield, P. J., Kleinhaus, K., Opler, M., Perrin, M., Learned, N., Goetz, R., Stanford, A., Messinger, J., Harkavy-Friedman, J., & Malaspina, D. (2010). Later paternal age and sex differences. *Schizophrenia Research 116*, 191–95.

Röttig, S., Wenzel, A., Blöink, R., & Brieger, P. (2004). Affective and schizoaffective mixed states. *European Archives of Psychiatry and Clinical Neuroscience 254*, 76–81.

Sandman, C. A., Glynn, L. M., & Davis, E. P. (2013). Is there a viability-vulnerability tradeoff? Sex differences in fetal programming. *Journal of Psychosomatic Research 75*, 327–35.

Schizophrenia Working Group of the Psychiatric Genomics Consortium. (2014). Biological insights from 108 schizophrenia-associated genetic loci. *Nature 511*, 421–27.

Schwartz, S, Meyer, IH. (2010). Mental health disparities research: The impact of within and between group analyses on tests of social stress hypotheses. *Social Science & Medicine. 70*, 1111–18.

Seeman, M. V. (1982). Gender differences in schizophrenia. *Canadian Journal of Psychiatry 27*, 107–12.

Seeman, M. V. (1989). Neuroleptic prescription for men and women. *Social Pharmacology 3*, 219–36.

Seeman, M. V. (2009a). Suicide among women with schizophrenia spectrum disorders. Journal of *Psychiatric Practice 15*, 235–42.

Seeman, M. V. (2009b). Mechanisms of sex differences: A historical perspective. *Journal of Women's Health 18*, 861–66.

Seeman, M. V. (2009c). Secondary effects of antipsychotics: Women at greater risk than men. *Schizophrenia Bulletin 35*, 937–48.

Seeman, M. V. (2010). Parenting issues in mothers with schizophrenia. *Current Women's Health Reviews 6*, 51–7.

Seeman, M. V. (2012a). Menstrual exacerbation of schizophrenia symptoms. *Acta Psychiatrica Scandinavica, 125*, 363–71.

Seeman, M. V. (2012b). Treating schizophrenia at the time of menopause. *Maturitas, 72*, 117–20.

Seeman, M. V. (2012c). Intervention to prevent child custody loss in mothers with schizophrenia. *Schizophrenia Research and Treatment, 2012*, 796763.

Seeman, M. V. (2013). Clinical interventions for women with schizophrenia: pregnancy. *Acta Psychiatrica Scandinavica, 127*, 12–22.

Seeman, M. V. (2015). Sexual minority women in treatment for serious mental illness - a literature review. *Journal of Gay & Lesbian Mental Health, 19*, 303–19.

Seeman, M. V., & Gupta, R. (2013). Selective review of age-related needs of women with schizophrenia. *Clinical Schizophrenia & Related Psychoses, 9*, 21–29.

Seeman, M. V., & Lang, M. (1990). The role of estrogens in schizophrenia gender differences. *Schizophrenia Bulletin 16*, 185–94.

Seeman, M. V., Ross, R. (2011). Prescribing contraceptives for women with schizophrenia. *Journal of Psychiatric Practice 17*, 258–69.

Sekar, A., Bialas, A. R., de Rivera, H., Davis, A., Hammond, T. R., Kamitaki, N., Tooley, K., Presumey, J., Baum, M., Van Doren, V., & Genovese, G. (2016). Schizophrenia risk from complex variation of complement component 4. *Nature, 530*, 177–83.

Smith, S. (2010). Gender differences in antipsychotic prescribing. *International Review of Psychiatry 22*, 472-484.

Sweeney, S., Air, T., Zannettino, L., & Galletly, C. (2015). Gender differences in the physical and psychological manifestation of childhood trauma and/or adversity in people with psychosis. *Frontiers in Psychology* doi: 10.3389/fpsyg.2015.01768.

Teplin, L.A. (1990). The prevalence of severe mental disorder among male urban jail detainees: Comparison with the Epidemiologic Catchment Area Program. *American Journal of Public Health 80*, 663–69.

Usall, J., Suarez, D., Haro, J.M., & SOHO Study Group. (2007). Gender differences in response to antipsychotic treatment in outpatients with schizophrenia. *Psychiatry Research 153*, 225–31.

van Reekum, R., Cohen, T., & Wong, J. (2000). Can traumatic brain injury cause psychiatric disorders? *Journal of Neuropsychiatry & Clinical Neuroscience 12*, 316–27.

Varese, F., Smeets, F., Drukker, M., Lieverse R., Lataster T., Viechtbauer W., Read, J., van Os, J., & Bentall, R. P. (2012). Childhood adversities increase the risk of psychosis: a meta-analysis of patient-control, prospective- and cross-sectional cohort studies. *Schizophrenia Bulletin 38*, 661–71.

Varner, F., & Mandara, J. (2013). Discrimination concerns and expectations as explanations for gendered socialization in African American families. *Child Development 84*, 875–90.

Waddell, A., Ross, L. Ladd, L., & Seeman, M. V. (2006). Safe Minds—Perceptions of safety in a rehabilitation clinic for serious persistent mental illness. *International Journal of Psychosocial Rehabilitation 11*, 4–10.

Weickert, T. W., Allen, K. M., & Weickert, C. S. (2016). Potential role of oestrogen modulation in the treatment of cognitive deficits in schizophrenia. *Central Nervous System Drugs 30*, 125–33.

Wells, J. C. (2000). Natural selection and sex differences in morbidity ad mortality in early life. *Journal of Theoretical Biology 202*, 65–76.

Wiers C. E., Shokri-Kojori E., Wong C. T., Abi-Dargham A., Demiral S. B., Tomasi D., Wang G.-Jm & Volkow N. D. Cannabis abusers show hypofrontality and blunted brain responses to a stimulant challenge in females but not in males. *Neuropsychopharmacology 41*, 2596–605.

Willhite, R. K., Niendam, T. A., Bearden, C. E., Zinberg, J., O'Brien, M. P., Cannon, T. D. (2008). Gender differences in symptoms, functioning and social support in patients at ultra-high risk for developing a psychotic disorder. *Schizophrenia Research 104*, 237–45.

Womer, F. Y., Tang, Y., Harms, M. P., Bai, C., Chang, M., Jiang, X., Wei, S., Wang, F., & Barch, D. M. (2016). Sexual dimorphism of the cerebellar vermis in schizophrenia. *Schizophrenia Research 176*, 164–70.

Yakushko, O., Watson, M., & Thompson, S. (2008). Stress and coping in the lives of recent immigrants and refugees: Considerations for counseling. *International Journal for the Advancement of Counselling 30*, 167–78.

Zilberman, M. L., Tavares, H., Blume, S. B., & el-Guebaly, N. (2003). Substance use disorders: Sex differences and psychiatric comorbidities. *Canadian Journal of Psychiatry 48*, 5–13.

Index

Abraham, N., 23, 32
abuse: case material, 28, 151–154; and
  eating disorders, 113–114;
  epidemiology, 166–167; by hospital
  staff, 176, 178; psychodynamic theory
  and, 113; and psychosis, 44, 113, 114,
  163–164, 166; schizophrenia and, 195.
  See also sexual abuse; trauma; cases:
  Alice; cases: Janet
Adair, M., 136
Alice in Wonderland (Carroll), 37
Angela of Foligno, 137
anorexia nervosa: antipsychotic
  medications and, 110; bulimia nervosa
  and, 111; case material, 114; child
  abuse and, 113, 114; feminism,
  feminists, and, 114, 116; psychiatric
  symptoms in, 111; psychodynamics,
  114–117; psychosis and, 110–113, 115
anorexic voice, 4, 111; stages in the
  development of, 111–112
Arieti, Silvano, 110, 115–117
art, 132. *See also* creativity
Asylums,. *See also* psychiatric ward(s);
  specific topics 19, 81, 90
Athan, A. A., 83, 97, 100
Atkinson, J., 22
attic, madwoman in the: in *Jane Eyre*,
  17–18, 40–42; *The Madwoman in the
  Attic* (Gilbert and Gubar), 40–43, 48
Austen Riggs Center, 23, 24, 31–32

Beatrice of Nazareth, 138
Beloved (Morrison), 48, 53–56
Beth: A Story of Postpartum Psychosis
  (Halvorson), 93–94
biopsychosocial model, 44
bipolar disorder, 164; case material, 25, 27,
  110, 175–176, 178; eating disorders
  and, 109; gender differences in,
  165–166; psychosis and, 44, 82, 87;
  postpartum, 81, 86–88, 91;
  schizophrenia and, 163–165
Bleuler, Eugen, 90
blind eye, turning a, 17
bodily ego, 114
body and mind, 15
body ego, 114
borderline personality disorder, 26–27, 163
Bordo, S., 114–115
Bourneville, Désiré-Magloire, 126, 132,
  134, 135, 144
Bowen, Elizabeth, 28–29
brain: gender differences in the, 167–168.
  See also neurology
brain pathology in schizophrenia, gender
  differences in, 167, 193
Bratton, M., 129
breastfeeding and postpartum psychosis,
  90
Bricquet, Pierre, 136
Brontë, Charlotte. *See also Jane Eyre* 17,
  41, 42

bulimia nervosa, 111, 113

cannabis abuse and schizophrenia, 191
Carey, Miriam, 94
cases: Alice, 173–176, 179, 180; Ava,
21–26, 31; Helen, 170–173, 179, 180;
Janet, 176–178; Kate, 27; Leah, 25–26;
Virginia, 27–28
Cassell, Eric J., 141
Cathars, 137
Catholic Church, 133, 142; *vs.* Cathars,
137; Charcot and, 132–133, 144;
Geneviève Basile Legrande and, 130,
131; hypnosis and, 133; hysteria and,
130–131, 133, 134; mysticism and, 133,
134, 137, 142–144; neurology and,
132–133; psychosis and, 130–132;
women and, 137, 142
Charcot, Jean-Martin, 131; art and, 130;
Catholic Church and, 132–133, 144;
diagnostic criteria and, 132; Geneviève
Basile Legrande and, 126, 132, 135,
139, 140, 144, 146; hysteria and,
130–136, 138, 139, 144, 146; life
history, 131; religion and, 132–134,
139, 144; at Salpêtrière, 126, 130, 135,
139, 140, 145; symptoms and, 131
Chermin, K., 114–115
Chesler, Phyllis, x, 19, 42
child abuse. *See* abuse; sexual abuse
childbirth, traumatic, 86, 87, 93, 98–100
Chödrön, Pema, 44
Christianity 137. *See also* Catholic Church
Claudel, Camille, 15
Cohen, K. D., 99
control, sense of, 84
"crazy"/craziness, designation of, 23,
28–30, 45–47, 156. *See also* literature:
"crazy" characters
creativity, 13, 21; psychosis and, 13, 23,
24, 27, 29, 30, 39
cultural devaluation 20. *See also*
sociocultural factors; implicated in
women's madness

de Lauretis, T., 14
delusions, 115; defined, 162. *See also*
specific topics

dementia praecox, 90, 164. *See also*
schizophrenia
depression, 87–89, 128; case material, 151,
152, 157, 173–175; of Gogo Ekhaya
Esima,. *See also* postpartum depression
151, 152, 157; psychosis and, 87, 111;
postpartum psychosis; postpartum
depression
Devereux, Cecily, 138–139
Didi-Huberman, Georges, 131
Dillon, Jacqui, 44
disabilities, 75; studies on, 57n1
discredited identities, x
dissociation, 113, 163
dissociative identity disorder. *See* multiple
personality disorder
The Divided Self (Laing), 45. *See also*
Laing, R. D.
dopamine, 168
drug abuse and schizophrenia, 190–191
dysregulation, 24, 27, 30. *See also* self-
regulation

eating disorders: child abuse, trauma, and,
113, 119; feminist analysis of, 114;
Hornbacher on, 115, 118;
Psychodynamics, 113–118; psychosis
and, 109, 111–116, 119; schizophrenia
and, 109–111, 117. *See also* anorexia
nervosa
ego boundaries, 96. *See also* self-other
boundaries
ego development, 114. *See also* identity
development
electroconvulsive therapy (ECT), 4, 69, 94,
100–101
Eliot, George, 16
Eliot, T. S., 59
embodied simulation, 16
emotional regulation. *See* dysregulation;
self-regulation
equilibrium, 21, 24; false self and, 44
estrogens, 165, 168
Euripides, 48, 51. *See also Medea*
externalization, 111, 114, 116, 119

false self, 55, 56; *Medea* and, 54; R. D.
Laing on, 45–46, 53

false-self system, 3, 44–46, 50; Andrea
    Yates and, 51; *Beloved* and, 54–56
feminism, 74; "white", 41
feminists, ix–x; of color, 43; on the
    diagnosis of "schizophrenia", x; on
    eating disorders, 114, 116; on hysteria,
    138, 141–142; and the literary
    madwoman, 38; on madness in women,
    42; postpartum psychosis and, 82, 98;
    on psychoanalysis, 126
Ferenczi, Sándor, 113
Forrest, W. C., 17
Fox, J. R., 111–112
fragmentation, vii, 30, 31, 113. *See also*
    identity diffusion; identity confusion
Freud, Sigmund, 13, 99
Frye, Northrop, 45, 46–47
Fulford, K. W., 129

Gallese, V., 16
Garcia, Adair, 95
Geertz, Clifford, 140–141
Geller, J. L., 19
gender differences: in the brain, 167–168;
    in expressions of illness, 166–168; in
    psychotic symptom profiles, 164–166;
    in schizophrenia, x, 187–195
Geneviève L. *See* Legrande, Geneviève
    Basile
Gilbert, Sandra, 40–43, 48
Gilman, Charlotte Perkins, 92
Gilman, S. L., 81
God, 129, 134, 138–141; mystical
    experiences and, 129; visions of, 129,
    143
Grosz, E., 85
Gubar, Susan, 40–43, 48

Hahn, Father, 133
hallucinations, 115–116, 162; defined, 162.
    See also anorexic voice; visions
Halvorson, Shirley Cervene, 93–94
Harris, M., 19
Hearing Voices Network Movement, 76
Hollywood, A. M., 137, 138
Hôpital Universitaire Pitié-Salpêtrière. *See*
    Salpêtrière
hormones: and the expression of illness,
    168; and the onset of illness, 168;

postpartum psychosis and, 83–85, 90,
    91, 192; and response to treatment,
    168–169
Hornbacher, M., 115, 118
Hornstein, G. A., 12
hospitals. *See* asylums; psychiatric ward(s)
Hustvedt, Asti, 128, 130. *See also*
    Legrande, Geneviève Basile
Hyman, Rebecca, 50, 51, 95
hypnosis, 133
hysteria, 139; as biological vulnerability in
    need of male interpretation, 5; Catholic
    Church and, 130–131, 133, 134;
    Charcot and, 130–136, 138, 139, 144,
    146; etiology, 136; feminist
    interpretations of, 138, 141–142;
    mysticism and, 126–127, 133, 134, 138,
    144, 145; psychosis, hysteria, and
    religion in context, 127–136, 145;
    Salpêtrière and, 134, 136–138; sex and,
    136, 143; stages in Charcot's model of,
    132; terminology, 132; treatment, 136;
    uses and meanings of the term,
    130–131. *See also* Legrande,
    Geneviève Basile
hysterical pregnancy, 142–143
hysterics, male, 136, 142

identities, "discredited", x
identity, split, 55. *See also* multiple
    personality disorder; splitting
identity development, 11, 21, 25, 113; case
    material, 25, 26, 28; in men, 15;
    narratives and, 31–32; parent-child
    relationship and, 11, 15, 20–22, 25, 26,
    31; and psychosis, 30; sociocultural
    oppression and, 11–12; women and, 11.
    See also false self; self-development
identity diffusion and identity confusion,
    31, 96, 97, 99. *See also* fragmentation;
    self-other boundaries
immunology and schizophrenia, 192
incest, 62, 63
infanticide, postpartum psychosis and,
    94–95
inner critic. *See* anorexic voice
insanity: (binary of) sanity *vs.*, 50, 92;
    terminology, 1, 38, 39. *See also* sanity;
    specific topics

insanity defense, 50
insight, lack of, 162
internalized oppression, 11, 14
internalized sexism, 114
internalized stigma, 88
internalized trauma, 22
intersectionality, 45

Jackson, Mike, 129
Jacques de Vitry, 137
Jane Eyre (Brontë), 17–18, 38, 41–42;
   madwoman (Bertha Mason) in, 18, 38,
   41–42
Jaspers, Karl, 90–91
Jesus Christ, 136
Jones, I., 88
Jones, N., 100

Karon, Bertram P., 98–99
Karraa, Walker, 94
Klompenhouwer, J., 89
Knapp, Caroline, 111, 114–116
Kraepelin, Emil, 90, 164
Krasner, Lee, 12
Kugelmann, R., 132

LaCapra, D., 11, 22
Laing, R. D., 45–46, 53, 70; and the
   madwoman, 45–46; and the true and
   false selves, 45–46, 53
Lateau, Louise, 125, 126, 132, 139, 140,
   142; Geneviève Basile Legrande and,
   125, 126, 132, 139, 140, 142
Lebow, J., 110
Lefebvre, Dr., 133
Legrande, Geneviève Basile, 125–126,
   128; background and early life,
   125–126, 128, 130; Catholic Church
   and, 130, 131, 142–144; depression
   and, 128; doctors, 126–128, 130, 134,
   140, 144, 145; Charcot, 126, 132, 135,
   140, 144; hysteria and, 125–127, 130,
   131, 134, 135, 139, 141–144; hysterical
   pregnancy, 142; Louise Lateau and,
   125, 126, 132, 139, 140, 142; psychosis
   and, 127–131; religion and, 130–131,
   133, 134, 139, 140–145; Salpêtrière
   and, 134, 140, 146; sexuality, 128, 130;
   suffering and self-interpretation,

139–145; treatment, 195; visions, 143,
   145
literary devices, 17
literary theme of the madwoman, 14, 38,
   43–44, 51, 56; reasons she appears, 44.
   See also Jane Eyre: madwoman (Bertha
   Mason) in; literature: "crazy"
   characters; minority identities
literature: "crazy" characters, 37–38, 43,
   45, 47; women and psychosis in, 16–18.
   See also literary theme of the
   madwoman; *specific literary works*
Lorde, Audre, 43, 59
Lyons, A., 102
"mad," etymology of the term, 39

madness: contextualizing, 19–20; stepping
   into, 48. *See also* psychosis; *specific*
   topics
madwoman: allure of the, 56; *The*
   Madwoman in the Attic (Gilbert and
   Gubar), 17–18, 42; R. D. Laing and the,
   45–46; and the true and false self, 46.
   See also literary theme of the
   madwoman; *specific topics*
Major Depressive Disorder, 82, 87
mania: postpartum psychosis and, 86, 89.
   See also postpartum psychosis; bipolar
   disorder
manic-depressive illness, 164. *See also*
   bipolar disorder
mansplaining, 44, 47
Marie d'Oignies, 137
marijuana abuse and schizophrenia, 190
Marzanski, M., 145
Mayman, Martin, 69–74
Mazzoni, C., 136, 144
McCarthy-Jones, Simon, 82
McWilliams, N., 97
Medea (Euripides), 48, 51–53
menstrual cycle, 165, 168
mental disabilities. *See* disabilities
metaphors, 31
minority identities, multiple: reading the
   madwoman to account for, 40–43
Morrison, Toni. *See Beloved*
Moyer, Jennifer Hentz, 92
multiple personality disorder (MPD), 26

mysticism: Catholic Church and, 132, 134, 137, 142; psychosis and, 138. *See also* mystics; spiritual experience and psychosis

mystics: Charcot and, 144, 145–146; erotic language of, 143; hysterics and, 126–127, 133, 134, 144, 145; medieval, x, 137–138, 143

negative symptoms, 59
neurasthenia, 136
neurology, 132–142. *See also* brain
neurotransmitter systems, 168, 192
nursing (breastfeeding) and postpartum psychosis, 61
nursing staff, 71, 177

object, use of an, 31
objectification: of oneself, 114, 117; of women, 13, 114, 117, 118. *See also* anorexia nervosa
Olson, M., x
Open Dialogue, ix, x
"other", 51, 59. *See also* self-other boundaries

Packard, Elizabeth, 15
pain and suffering, 141. *See also* suffering
Palazzoli, M. S., 109, 117
parent-child relationship, 100; and identity development, 11, 15, 20–22, 25, 26, 31
patriarchy, x
perceptualization of the concept, 116
Pitié-Salpêtrière Hospital. *See* Salpêtrière
possession, spirit, 49, 95, 130, 132, 136
postpartum depression, 83–84; Andrea Yates and, 50; compared with postpartum psychosis, 106n1; *DSM* and, 50, 58n3; epidemiology, 58n3; Miriam Carey and, 94
postpartum psychosis (PP), 3, 81, 82, 84, 86, 90, 103; compared with postpartum depression, 106n1; conceptions of and discourse on, 83, 86; diagnosis, 87–88; as diagnostic category, 50; *DSM* and, 50, 58n3; early feminist interpretations of, 98; epidemiology and risk factors, 85–86, 106n1; etiology of, 83; functional explanations, 84; hormonal

theories, 83–85, 90–91, 192; feminists and, 82, 83, 98; first-person accounts, 92–94; historical perspectives, 90–91; infanticide and, 94–95; psychoanalysis and, 82, 98–99; recovery, 102; schizophrenia and, 89, 96, 98; self-disturbance and, 96–97; sexuality and, 90, 97; spirituality and, 100; symptoms, 89; treatments for, 84, 100–101; barriers to the development of psychological, 101; writings on, 82, 83, 98, 99

pregnancy, hysterical, 142
premenstrual syndrome (PMS), 83, 97
pre-psychotic panic, 116
psychiatric ward(s): staff experience at, 181–182; women's experiences of the, 180–181. *See also* asylums; *specific topics*
psychiatry: research perspectives within, 164–167. *See also specific topics*
psychoanalysis, 11, 29; hysteria and, 141–142; psychosis and, 29; postpartum, 82, 97–98; sexism and phallocentrism in, 13, 141–142; women and, 14, 24, 42
psychoanalytic interpretation of visions, 143–144
psychoanalytic psychotherapy, 24, 26, 29, 31
psychosis: "colorful personalities" and, 30; definitions, 116, 127–128, 162–164; etymology of the term, 39; phases in the development of, 116; understandings of the term within psychiatry, 162–164; variability in, 43–44; clinical context, 21–28; documentaries on, 14. *See also* madness; *specific topics*
psychotic break, 116–117
"psychotic," use of the term, 162–164
puerperal mania, 81, 85. *See also* postpartum psychosis

Quindlen, Anna, 49

rape. *See* sexual assault
Read, John, 44
recognition scenes, 46

reflective capacity and reflective functioning, 19, 29, 30, 164; defined, 19

religion, 145; Charcot and, 132–134, 139, 144; defining, 134; Geneviève Basile Legrande and, 130–132, 138, 140, 140–141; *vs.* psychiatry, 127; psychosis, hysteria, and, 127–135, 145; Salpêtrière and, 134, 135, 136–139, 145; "true", 134, 139. *See also* Catholic Church; mystics

resistance, 23, 47; to hearing the true self, 50; madness as, 41

Rhys, Jean, 18, 27

Richer, Paul, 143

Robertson, E., 102

Rosenberg, 98

Roth, N., 99

Salpêtrière: Charcot at, 125, 130, 131, 135, 139, 140, 145; Geneviève Basile Legrande and, 134, 140, 146; hysteria and, 134, 136–138, 145; religion and, 134, 135, 136–139, 145

"sane", 39, 45

Sangoma, 155–157

sanity, 15, 19, 39. *See also* insanity; *specific topics*

schizoid persons, 113, 115

schizophrenia, 195; bipolar disorder and, 165; diagnosis of, x, 28, 43, 127, 176; eating disorders and, 109–111, 117; gender differences in, 187, 195; age of onset, 166, 168; brain pathology, 167, 193; clinical features, x, 188–190; epidemiology, 187–188; hormonal explanatory mechanisms, 192; prevention and treatment, 193–195; risk factors, 190–191; historical perspective on, 164; overview, 43; postpartum psychosis and, 86, 89, 90, 98; self-disturbance and, 96; symptoms, x, 127, 187–189

Searles, Harold F., 109, 117

Seeman, Mary V., 112

Seikkula, J., x

self, false *vs.* true. *See* false self

self-abnegation, 16, 22

self-agency and recovery from psychosis, 83

self-development, 20, 22, 25, 31. *See also* identity development

self-disturbance and psychosis, 96–97

self-fragmentation. *See* fragmentation

self-hatred, 11

self-other boundaries, 59, 92, 96–97, 129. *See also* identity diffusion and identity confusion

self-regulation, 113. *See also* dysregulation

sex-role alienation, x

sexual abuse, 28, 63, 115, 166, 168, 177, 190, 194

sexual assault, 70–71, 151

sexual behavior: case material, 174; delusions related to, 115

sexuality, vii–ix, 59, 68, 131; eating disorders and, 111, 113; hysteria and, 136, 143; mysticism and, 143, 144; postpartum psychosis and, 82, 90

sexual orientation, 69

sexual visions, 126, 127–131, 139, 142–143

shadow, 41–42

shamanic illness, 155

shamanic initiation, 155–157

shamanism, 155

shame, 4, 11, 23, 30, 63, 64, 115

Showalter, Elain, 90, 95, 136, 142

Smith, S., 88

social inclusion, 172

sociocultural factors implicated in women's madness, 13–16, 117–118

Solnit, Rebecca, 2, 38, 44, 47

Somé, Malidoma Patrice, 155

Soteria, 70

South Africa, 155–157

Spinoza, Baruch, 134

spirit possession, 49, 95, 130, 136

spiritual awakening/emergence and psychosis, 100, 156

"Spiritual Experience and Psychopathology" (Jackson and Fulford), 129

spiritual experience and psychosis, 129–130, 137. *See also* Legrande, Geneviève Basile; mysticism and psychosis; mystics

splitting, 41, 55, 119. *See also* identity
structural trauma, 11, 22
substance abuse and schizophrenia,
190–191
suffering, 100, 141; defined, 141. *See also*
Legrande, Geneviève Basile
Suicidality, 50, 51; postpartum psychosis
and, 50, 93
suicide attempts, 50, 140, 153
superstition *vs.* true religion, 134

Teresa of Ávila, 133
thought disorder, 162
Tierney, S., 111–112
Tovino, S. A., 90
trauma, 12, 26, 30, 113; case material, 28,
152, 156; and eating disorders, 113,
119; gender differences in, 190;
interpersonal, 113; and psychosis, 19,
22, 26, 28, 31, 43, 86, 113, 119,
163–164, 166; structural/generalized,
11, 22. *See also* abuse
traumatic childbirth, 86, 93, 98–100
trauma trails, 22
true self, resistance to hearing the, 50
true-self system. *See* false-self system
Tunnell, A., 118

turning a blind eye to difficult meanings,
17
Twomey, Teresa M., 95–96

use of an object, 31
Ussher, Jane M., x, 82, 83, 106n1

Van Gogh, Vincent, 30
Varner, Lynne, 95
visions: Geneviève's religious, 126,
128–129, 139, 142, 143; Geneviève's
sexual, 126, 128–129, 143–145

Wilner, Eleanor, 52–53
Winnicott, Donald W., 31, 97, 100
witch(es), viii, ix; madwoman as, 14
witch hunts, 130
womb: Hippocratic tradition and the, 135;
hysteria and the, 4–5, 135–136, 141
Women and Madness (Chesler), 19, 42. *See
also* Chesler, Phyllis
Woolf, Virginia, ix, 16, 30

Yates, Andrea, 49–51, 55, 95
"The Yellow Wallpaper" (Gilman), 92

Ziedoris, D., x
Zilboorg, Gregory, 98

About the Editors and Contributors

Marie Brown, MA is a clinical psychology doctoral candidate at Long Island University Brooklyn and a co-founder of Hearing Voices Network New York City. She is an active member of the U.S. chapter of the International Society for Psychological & Social Approaches to Psychosis (ISPS-US) and chair of the ISPS Special Interest Group on Psychosocial Factors in Postpartum Psychosis. Along with Marilyn Charles, she is co-chair of the American Psychological Association (APA) Division 39 (Psychoanalysis) Task Force on Psychosis & Dissociation. She holds a strong commitment to promoting co-led and collaborative research between people with lived experience and clinical researchers.

Marilyn Charles, PhD is a staff psychologist at the Austen Riggs Center and a psychoanalyst in private practice in Stockbridge, MA. Her research interests include creativity, psychosis, resilience, and the intergenerational transmission of trauma. She serves as contributing editor of *Psychoanalysis, Culture, and Society* and has presented her work internationally, publishing over 100 articles and book chapters and ten books: *Patterns: Building Blocks of Experience*, *Constructing Realities: Transformations Through Myth and Metaphor*, *Learning from Experience: a Guidebook for Clinicians*, *Working with Trauma: Lessons from Bion and Lacan*, *Psychoanalysis and Literature: The Stories We Live*, and (with co-editor Michael O'Loughlin) *Fragments of Trauma and the Social Production of Suffering*.

Jessica Arenella, PhD is a clinical psychologist in private practice in New York and New Jersey and has worked with people experiencing extreme and unusual experiences for two decades in a variety of settings. She is a co-founder of Hearing Voices Network New York City. Dr. Arenella currently serves as the president of the U.S. chapter of the International Society for Psychological and Social Approaches to Psychosis (ISPS-US).

Berta Britz, MSW, ACSW, CPS is a member of the Experts by Experience Committee of ISPS-US. Her ministry, "Hearing Voices and Healing," is under the care of Central Philadelphia Monthly Meeting of the Religious Society of Friends. She worked for over nine years in Montgomery County, Pennsylvania at Creating Increased Connections. As a certified Peer specialist, she was instrumental in introducing the Hearing Voices Movement to Montgomery County and has coordinated the Montgomery County Hearing Voices Network (www.mchvn.org). A board member of HVN-USA, Berta is an experienced facilitator of Hearing Voices Network Groups and has presented in many venues in the United States and internationally. She uses the liberation she experienced in the international Hearing Voices community to inform collaboration among mental health clinicians, family members and people with lived anomalous experiences to grow capacity for understanding the experience of living and working with anomalous beliefs and voices. Her deepest passion is for creating spaces that welcome young people growing into their fullest selves. She offers consultation and training through Berta Britz Consulting.

Nicola Byrne, MBChB, BSc, MSc, MRCPsych is a consultant psychiatrist and deputy medical director at the South London and Maudsley NHS Foundation Trust in London. She has worked in both community and inpatient mental health settings, and for the last ten years has been a consultant on an inpatient unit for women in Lambeth, south London. She is also chair of the UK's Royal College of Psychiatrists "Women and Mental Health" group.

Liane F. Carlson, PhD is the Stewart Postdoctoral Fellow and lecturer in Religion at Princeton University. received her PhD in philosophy of religion at Columbia University in 2015, where she received her M.A. (2010) and M.Phil (2012) after graduating summa cum laude from Washington and Lee University (2007). Her research interests include the philosophical and theological history of Critical Theory, with particular emphasis theories of religion, the limits of the critical power of history, embodiment, evil, and the intersection of religion and literature. Liane's work has been supported by a Fulbright Grant, a Jacob K. Javits Doctoral Fellowship, an AAUW American Dissertation Fellowship, a Mellon Interdisciplinary Graduate Fellowship, and a Public Humanities Fellowship from the New York Council for the Humanities.

Simone Ciufolini MD, PhD is a psychiatrist, psychotherapist, and researcher at the Institute of Psychiatry, Psychology and Neurology, King's College

London. He is a member of the Royal College of Psychiatrist and the Refugee Resilience Collective. Simone is interested in understanding how the interactions between environmental influences and individual characteristics interact to shape our human experience as well as the disease psychopathology. He is studying with the role that childhood trauma, stress response, and gender have in the neurobiology underlying mental health, psychosis in particular.

Helen DeVinney, PsyD is a member of the core faculty at The George Washington University Professional Psychology Program, where she teaches doctoral classes in psychodynamic psychopathology, gender development, and clinical psychotherapy. Helen pursued training in a psychoanalytically-informed doctoral program after first completing graduate work in English and Critical Theory. She holds advanced degrees in Teaching, English, and Psychology. She is particularly interested in working with and thinking about dissociation as well as the intersections of psychoanalysis and issues of gender, sexuality, race, class, ability, and complex trauma. Helen has a private practice in Washington, D.C. where she provides therapy, assessment, and supervision.

Gogo Ekhaya Esima is an initiated Sangoma traditional healer in the Zulu culture of South Africa. She is a certified Peer recovery specialist in mental health, a trauma survivor, and a spiritual teacher. She is as strong advocate for challenging standardized mental health concepts in America and her shamanic journey of healing and recovery is featured in the documentary CRA-ZYWISE. Her gifts include seeing and hearing voices of the ancestors, mediumship, and earth-based medicinal healing. Gogo Ekhaya has a full-time shamanic healing practice in Southern California. www.sangomahealing.com

Mary V. Seeman, MD is professor Emerita, Department of Psychiatry, University of Toronto. Her lifelong interest has been in the effect of psychosis on women and the effect of gender on psychosis. Dr. Seeman has written over 350 scientific articles and authored several books. She has served as psychiatrist-in-chief at Mt. Sinai Hospital and as vice-chair of the University of Toronto Department of Psychiatry, as well as inaugural Tapscott Professor and Chair of Schizophrenia Studies. She has received an honorary degree from the University of Toronto, and has been inducted as an officer into the Order of Canada for her contributions to the mental health of Canadian women.